Practical Diet Guide to Intermittent Fasting For Women Over 50

Fast Track Success: The Weight Loss Diet Plan That Tackles Inflammation & Boosts Mind and Body for a Healthier, Longer Life

Julia Bennett

Mindful Insights

Copyright © 2024 by Julia Bennett/Goldberry Hill.

All rights reserved.

The content contained within this book may not be reproduced, duplicated or transmitted without direct written permission from the author or the publisher. No part of this book may be reproduced in any form or by any electronic or mechanical means, including information storage and retrieval systems, without written permission from the author, except for the use of brief quotations in a book review.

Under no circumstances will any blame or legal responsibility be held against the publisher, or author, for any damages, reparation, or monetary loss due to the information contained within this book. Either directly or indirectly. You are responsible for your own choices, actions, and results.

Legal Notice:

This book is copyright protected. This book is only for personal use. You cannot amend, distribute, sell, use, quote or paraphrase any part, or the content within this book, without the consent of the author or publisher.

Disclaimer Notice:

Please note the information contained within this document is for educational and entertainment purposes only. All effort has been executed to present accurate, up to date, and reliable, complete information. No warranties of any kind are declared or implied. Readers acknowledge that the author is not engaging in the rendering of legal, financial, medical or professional advice. The content within this book has been derived from various sources. Please consult a licensed professional before attempting any techniques outlined in this book.

By reading this document, the reader agrees that under no circumstances is the author responsible for any losses, direct or indirect, which are incurred as a result of the use of the information contained within this document, including, but not limited to, errors, omissions, or inaccuracies.

Contents

Introduction	vii
1. LET'S BEGIN	1
What is Intermittent Fasting	2
Men and Women	3
Why We Diet and Pitfalls of Other Diets	3
What are we targetting	6
Insulin	6
Cortisol	7
Metabolic Rate	8
2. INFLAMMATION AND INTERMITTENT FASTING	9
Cytokines and CRP	9
Cholesterol Levels	10
Oxidative Stress and Free Radicals	11
Key Takeaways So Far	12
3. METABOLIC RATE & METABOLIC SWITCHING	14
Understanding Metabolic Rate	14
Basal Metabolic Rate (BMR)	14
Resting Metabolic Rate (RMR)	15
Thermic Effect of Food (TEF)	15
Physical Activity	15
Adaptive Thermogenesis	15
Energy Balance	16
Metabolic Flexibility	16
Autophagy & mTOR	18
Ketones and Cancer	19
Ketosis	20
Hormetic Stress	20
Symptoms (or problems or solve)	21
Intermittent Fasting	21
Excessive Fasting	22

Signs of Poor or Weak Metabolic Health	24
Tips and Tools	27
4. EXERCISES	**28**
Quiz	28
Exercises	32
Metabolic Switching Symptom Tracker	33
5. WHAT NOT TO EAT	**38**
Foods Low in Calories but Also Low in Nutrients	39
Common Obesogens and Their Sources	42
Identifying Exposure Obesogens	46
Synthetic Ingredients Found in Common Foods	48
Actions to minimise exposure to Obesogens	50
Foods to Avoid	51
6. GLYCEMIC LOAD MATTERS	**52**
Categories of Glycemic Index	53
Low GI Foods (55 or less)	53
Medium GI Foods (56-69)	56
High GI Foods (70 and above)	58
Tips for Managing Glycemic Index	60
Planning an intermittent fasting diet with GI and nutrients	61
7. FOODS TO EAT	**67**
Role of Cofactors in Cellular Functions	67
The Role of Nutrients in Cellular Functions	68
Energy Production	69
Glucose Metabolism	69
Antioxidant Production and Function	69
Reminder: Nutrient Balance and Why It Works	70
Key Vitamins and Why They're Important	70
Healthy Fats	71
Quality Proteins	71
Nutrient-dense foods	72
Antioxidants	74
Plan a Day's Meal Incorporating Nutrient-Dense Foods	75
Getting started	76

Exercise	77
Before you begin: Exercises and Reflective Questions	78
8. EXAMPLE MENU	**84**
Example Daily Diet	84
9. GOALS AND FASTING TYPES	**102**
What is your goal?	104
Type of Fast	105
10. WOMEN, HORMONES AND GLUCOSE	**113**
Action Plans	115
Menopause and Beyond	117
Action Plans	119
11. MEN, HORMONES AND ANDROPAUSE	**121**
Common Symptoms and Conditions	121
12. FASTING PLANNING	**125**
Ending a Fast	126
Action Plans	127
Goal Setting	128
Action Plans example	129
13. THE 12:12 KICK-START 30-DAY PLAN	**147**
Daily Structure	148
Week 1: Getting Started (Days 1-7)	148
Week 2: Incorporating Variety (Days 8-14)	149
Week 3: Maintaining Momentum (Days 15-21)	150
Week 4: Continuing Healthy Habits (Days 22-28)	151
Week 5: Final Week and Adjustments (Days 29-30)	152
Breaking the Fast: Tips and Adjustments	153
Key Nutrients and Their Importance	153
14. MOVING UP TO 16:8 30 DAY PLAN	**155**
Week 1: Getting Started (Days 1-7)	156
Week 2: Incorporating Variety (Days 8-14)	156
Week 3: Maintaining Momentum (Days 15-21)	156
Week 4: Continuing Healthy Habits (Days 22-28)	157
Week 5: Final Week and Adjustments (Days 29-30)	157

15. RECIPES	158
Recipes	158
16. YOUR FASTING LIFESTYLE	170
Recommended Exercises	170
Under 50	170
Women Over 50	171
Men Over 50	172
Practical Implementation and Benefits	173
Other Lifestyle Practices	174
Stress Reduction	174
Adequate Sleep	175
Proper Hydration	175
Mindful Eating	177
Goal Setting	178
Chapter Summary	178
Action Plan examples to support goals	181
17. PRACTICAL TIPS AND TRICKS	183
Managing Hunger During Fasting	183
Beverage Choices While Fasting	184
Handling Detox Symptoms	184
Monitoring Blood Sugar and Ketones	184
Fasting and Specific Conditions	185
Fatigue and Sleep	186
Overcoming Challenges in Fasting	187
Goal Setting	190
Action Plans	191
Getting Started	193
18. 5 KEY GOALS	194
5 Short Term Goals	194
5 Long-term Goals	195
19. ACTION PLANS	196
20. BEGINNER FASTING LOGS	201
Weekly beginner logs	211
21. CONCLUSION	227
22. REFERENCES	229

Introduction

For some reason, us humans, seems to have an aversion to doing things that are good for us - or at the very least, we find them difficult to start and then harder to keep the momentum going. This includes exercise, taking time out, or not starting a healthy diet.

For me, the hurdle was often too much information so that I had volumes of it. This led to seminars and courses, limiting my time (or so I told myself) so that I had no time to work out a simple path that told me exactly what I needed to do and which I could start right away. Or which helped me to remember what to do each day, while I got used to it all.

It goes without saying that how we think about ourselves matters and that everything begins by realising that we are worth the effort, that we are allowed to love ourselves and that self love incudes loving and taking care of our bodies and our mind. The other part of the barrier is realising that we are all responsible for our actions and outcomes, and taking responsibility is often more than half the battle. This can, of course, mean taking responsibility for providing ourselves with love.

Introduction

When I began this journey I knew that I wanted to be healthier, fitter and have more energy and focus. I also knew how important diet was and is, not only to weight, but for mental and long term general health. As ever, both my physical and digital shelf was full of books on intermittent fasting and I decided to write a book for myself, to write the book I needed to get started, and that reminded me of what and why I was doing the things I needed to do. And I needed something practical - I needed to somehow imbed and remember what I knew.

Luckily I had already done a workbook on this very subject - and this is what this book is based around. It focuses on the key things you need to know and remember, with planners and exercises. The aim is simply to start and stick to it for 30 days. If you do this, then you can move on to exploring different goals that fasting can help with, already knowing which food you love, why you need it, and with the confidence of knowing that it will work.

I am now over 50, and so I was well aware that I needed to take account of my hormone levels (I also know an awful lot about women's health having previously written about it) and so I had to think about the information that I needed to account for this.

I then sat down with all my own work on health, from menopause and herbs to the vagus nerve, and re-read and re-visited my bookshelves, favourite authors and courses, and I wrote this book.

Before we get started on all the detail what follows is a very brief summary of how and why it all works.

Unsurprisingly our body, which means our cells, needs glucose for energy. Our gut takes the food and extracts the energy it contains and this energy gets transferred around our body with the help of insulin. In even simpler terms, glucose cannot enter our cells without the help of insulin.

When insulin levels fall, it stimulates us to eat more food so that it can get its 'food energy' which is one of the reason we feel hungry.

Introduction

Now, if our body can't get the glucose, it waits for 4 or 5 hours before making us feel hungry to replenish the energy and if it isn't forthcoming then it will find other energy sources, which involves a little bit more work and uses a bit more energy.

Usually, it waits for around 8 hours before it takes this action. It will then stop producing insulin and switch to glucagon which stimulates our liver to release its store of glycogen which it can break down into glucose. This will last for around 6 hours.

Once this runs out, your body has yet another option, and it's fat. And this is what is known as Ketosis i.e. when our body starts to use fat for energy. This takes place after the glucose for food and the supply from the liver has run out (around 14 hours after eating, but it can be a little longer for some people). These fat cells are a much better source of glucose for your brain, which is why it can help 'brain fog' - and, it helps you lose weight. In a very simple nutshell, that is intermittent fasting!

I am happy to report that my fasting is working for me and my energy and focus levels are beyond what I had expected. I hope that you, too, find it useful and that it gives you the nudge you need to begin trying it out, or even simply to pique your interest so that you go on to find out more. Or even, get to know more about the food that our bodies need.

Chapter 1

Let's Begin

Intermittent fasting is not a new concept. It goes back to the beginning of our hunter-gatherer ancestry, but it's only in the last few years that it has gained momentum again, thanks, in part, to the Keto diet and books such as Fast Like a Girl.

Our ancestors often experienced periods of food scarcity and naturally adapted to cycles of fasting and feasting based on the availability of food, and this historical pattern is reflected in modern intermittent fasting practices, where people cycle between periods of eating and fasting to potentially improve health and manage weight.

While the Keto diet has contributed to the trend by promoting similar metabolic effects, intermittent fasting has also gained attention through various scientific studies highlighting its potential health benefits, as well as improved metabolic health, it as been shown to reduce inflammation, enhance cognitive function and even benefit longevity. And all of these are the scourge of anyone over 50.

It means that intermittent fasting isn't only a diet about weight management - it can be - but it doesn't need to be. This is because it has a host of other health improvements beyond weight loss, particularly those of us who have grown into our 50's and beyond.

It's also very much to do with mindset - and your personal goals and your personal plan. It means that understanding yourself and your body is perhaps the most important tool in your box which will help you achieve that which you know you can, and that which you know you want to. To do all of this, you need to know about what's going on. It's the only way that I can persuade you to give it go.

What is Intermittent Fasting

Intermittent fasting simply means taking a pause from eating to let you body rest and repair. In other words, you have an eating period and a fasting period. The easiest method is what is the 12:12 all the to what is called the 16:8. In the case of the 16:8 it means eating for 8 hours and not eating for 16 hours. For example, you can eat between 10am and 6pm or noon until 8pm or any variation - as long as you have an 8 hour eating window and don't eat at all for the remaining 16 hours of the day.

If that worries you, then that's why you will be pleased to know that the best place to start is a 12:12 - 12 hours of rest and 12 hours of eating. You can start there - or stay there - it will help even if you don't want to move up to longer fast lengths like the 16:8.

Other popular methods are called the 5:2, you eat for 5 days and pause for 2, or alternate day fasting when you eat one day, and don't eat the next day. We won't go into detail on these here - the aim is to get started and make it as easy as possible to start reaping the many rewards. Fasting for more than 36 hours might also not be great if you are over 50 and some doctors would advise against fasts lasting any longer than this. We'll cover this later in the book but its to do with your hormones and muscle mass.

You also don't even need to do this every day or week of the year, and learning how to break a fast is just as important as fasting itself. For women not already in menopause and still regularly cycling, or pregnant, then there are times when it's better not to fast at all. We'll cover both of these in the following pages.

But before we get into the details, let's talk about three important factors in weight management, diets and health general: insulin, cortisol, and metabolic rate (which come up again and again in later chapters) as well as the difference between intermittent fasting and traditional diets.

Men and Women

First of all, if you live with someone then the success of an eating plan, especially when it comes to food, shopping and cooking is often higher when you can both take part and enjoy it together. Men also experience changes as they age and while most nutrients are the same between men and women, there are some variations that can help one or the other specifically. It means that an intermittent fasting diet can work for both sexes and, with small adjustments, the same plates of food can be served which target the different needs of woman depending on the ovulatory cycle or age, and men dealing with declining testosterone and other vitamins as they also age. While the following pages do focus primarily on women, men aren't forgotten!

Why We Diet and Pitfalls of Other Diets

Even before we talk about the intermittent fasting diet, it's worthwhile taking a look at the 'traditional diets', and why it's not your fault that they might not always work for you.

Calorie-counting diets work by having you keep track of how many calories you eat. The idea is to eat fewer calories than your body needs, so it has to use up stored calories to get the energy it needs. Your body turns these calories into something called ATP, which is type of the energy your cells need use to work. Your body stores energy in the form of both fat and carbohydrates (like glycogen in your muscles and liver). When you eat fewer calories, your body starts to use these stored forms of energy.

The thinking is that by reducing this fuel, our bodies will use our 'stored' calories to generate the energy we need each day, and this helps us lose weight. Nothing wrong with that, you might think. And for some people, this is exactly how it works, but for many, if not most of us, it doesn't.

Don't take my word for it. According to the Institute of Diabetes and Digestive and Kidney Diseases (NIDDK), the calorie restriction approach can alter the body's metabolic set-point, making sustainable weight management difficult and we'll talk more about this is Chapter 3 and later in this chapter. On top of that, when calorie intake is drastically reduced, the body can even respond by slowing down metabolism, making it harder to lose weight and easier to regain it.

Extreme calorie restriction can also lead to nutrient deficiencies, because rigid diet plans can ignore our unique differences in metabolism and personal health needs. The National Institutes of Health (NIH) says that our cells require a variety of nutrients to produce energy (ATP), metabolise glucose, and to create antioxidants that fight oxidative stress. A diet needs to be nutrient-rich to help maintain these processes, which in turn supports overall bodily function and performance. Nutrients such as vitamins, minerals, and antioxidants play critical roles in these cellular functions and, of course, our overall health.

It means that 'traditional diets', by their very nature, can be too restrictive, nutritionally imbalanced, or simply not suited to individual needs. In other words, our body needs nutritional quality rather than just calorie counting. And because they are not sustainable nor aligned with how our bodies work, they fail. Don't blame yourself; your body is doing its job.

The other problem with these diets is that they can be hard to stick to. Cutting out carbs or fat can make you feel deprived, and you might end up craving the foods you're trying to avoid. On top of this, once you stop the diet, it's easy to go back to old eating habits and regain the weight.

This is where intermittent fasting comes with its focus on when you eat, not what you eat. You cycle between periods of eating and fasting helping you to eat fewer calories without having to cut out specific foods, and your body still uses stored energy during the fasting periods. Having said that, and as already mentioned, nutrients matter to our health, particularly as we age. This is why what we really should be eating is a big part of this book because it means we can live longer and be healthier as we do - allowing us to enjoy ourselves for a long time to come.

Now, returning to an important part of the jigsaw: your body has something called a metabolic set-point. This is like a thermostat for your weight. Your body likes to stay within a certain weight range, and it will adjust things like your hunger and energy levels to keep you there. When you diet, your body might slow down your metabolism to save energy, making it harder to lose weight and easier to gain it back once you stop dieting.

Intermittent fasting might help with this because it can improve your metabolic health. It can help your body become more efficient at using energy and can even help reset your metabolic set-point to a lower weight. This means you might not feel as hungry, because your body won't fight as hard to regain the weight you lost.

Mental health is also a big part of this. Stress can have a huge impact on your weight and overall health - including inflammation. High stress levels can mess with your hormones, making you hungrier and more likely to store fat. By giving your digestive system regular breaks, it has a calming effect on your body, and helps reduce stress.

Your vagus nerve, which runs from your brain to your gut, plays a role here too by managing this stress and inflammation. Fasting can help improve the function of the vagus nerve, leading to better stress management and lower inflammation levels. This, in turn, can improve your overall mental health and make you feel more balanced. Inflammation is a favourite topic of mine because it impacts so much of our health, so don't ever think that managing and looking after inflammation is a side issue.

Gut health too, is connected to both Vagal health and the positive impact of intermittent fasting, and a healthy gut can reduce inflammation and improve your mood. Intermittent fasting can literally give your gut time to rest and repair, leading to a healthier gut microbiome. Once again, this can reduce inflammation in your body and improve your mental health - a healthy gut is linked to better mood and lower levels of anxiety and depression.

So, while traditional diets can be tough and sometimes work against your body's natural tendencies, intermittent fasting offers a different approach that might be easier to maintain and better for long-term weight management, mental health, overall health and longevity.

What are we targetting

Insulin

As we have mentioned, insulin is the hormone that helps your body use glucose (sugar) from the food you eat. When you eat, your blood sugar levels rise, prompting your pancreas to release insulin to enable your cells to absorb this glucose for energy.

Today, our diets tend to be high in sugar, processed foods - or both - and this can lead to insulin resistance. Frequent spikes in blood sugar and corresponding high insulin levels can also overwhelm the body's cells, leading them to become less responsive to insulin. It means our cells are prevented from doing their glucose absorption job effectively and this excess glu. cose is stored as fat. This is what leads to weight gain and increasing the risk of type 2 diabetes as well as some other metabolic disorders. Inflammation can also interfere with the normal function of our insulin signalling which can also disrupt the ability of cells to respond to insulin effectively. To add insult to injury, visceral fat can lead to inflammation too.

Cortisol

Cortisol, often called the stress hormone, is released by your adrenal glands during stressful situations. While it's essential for your body's response to stress, chronic stress can lead to consistently high levels of cortisol. Elevated cortisol levels can increase blood sugar levels and also interfere with insulin, increasing fat storage, especially around the belly. This not only hampers weight loss but also affects your overall well-being.

Visceral fat, the fat stored around internal organs in the abdominal area, is particularly sensitive to the effects of high cortisol levels and lead to a greater accumulation of fat in this region. Visceral fat is not just a storage issue; it can also cause inflammation, which contributes to insulin resistance.

And, of course, when our insulin pathways are disrupted and our cells become less responsive to insulin, it leads to the body storing even more fat around the abdomen. This cycle of increased fat storage and insulin resistance can make any metabolic health issues worse.

Metabolic Rate

Your metabolic rate, which we have touched on, and go on to talk about in more detail, is the rate at which your body burns calories to maintain basic bodily functions, such as breathing and digestion. Even at rest all of these can help with weight loss. Factors like age, muscle mass, and genetics influence your metabolic rate while doing some regular physical activity, building muscle, and eating nutrient-dense foods can help your metabolism.

Along with metabolic rate, we have autophagy and mTOR which we cover these in chapter 3.

The next few chapters deal will deal in more detail with what we have touched on here. I would recommend that you read and try to understand this so that you know the benefits of what you are doing as you fast. You can skip this and go straight to the types of fast if you like, and come back to the science later.

However, next we have inflammation and this is one of the biggest upsides for anyone over 50.

Chapter 2

Inflammation and Intermittent Fasting

The anti-inflammatory benefits of intermittent fasting are among my favorites. It basically provides the body with the time it needs to engage in repair and maintenance activities, leading to these wide-ranging health benefits which we discuss in this chapter. Don't forget, chronic inflammation can lead to conditions such as arthritis, diabetes, and heart disease.

Cytokines and CRP

When you practice intermittent fasting, your body produces fewer pro-inflammatory cytokines, which are small proteins that can cause inflammation. Cytokines play a crucial role in controlling the immune response, inflammation, and the creation of blood cells. They work by attaching to specific receptors on target cells, triggering processes that change the behavior of those cells.

Studies have shown that both intermittent fasting and prolonged fasting (fasts lasting more than 24 hours) can significantly decrease levels of inflammatory markers like C-reactive protein (CRP) -

commonly measured in blood tests. CRP is a substance produced by the liver in response to inflammation and it is classified as an 'acute-phase protein', meaning its levels rise rapidly in response to inflammation or infection. CRP is a marker that doctors measure to assess inflammation in the body, and high levels of CRP indicate higher inflammation.

While cytokines are produced by various cells, including immune cells, it is mainly produced by the liver. Because insulin helps control blood sugar levels and with the liver playing a crucial role in this process, when insulin sensitivity improves, the liver gets better at regulating glucose levels and this reduces the production of these inflammatory molecules.

As you will discover in the next chapter, intermittent fasting improves autophagy which can reduces chronic inflammation, helping healthier liver function.

Cholesterol Levels

Intermittent fasting also improves cholesterol levels, particularly by lowering LDL ("bad" cholesterol) and increasing HDL ("good" cholesterol). Lower LDL levels mean less cholesterol buildup in the arteries, which reduces the risk of atherosclerosis (hardening of the arteries). Since high cholesterol is linked to increased inflammation and heart disease, better cholesterol levels contribute to reduced inflammation and improved heart health.

It means that intermittent fasting can improve heart health by lowering blood pressure and cholesterol levels, and since heart disease is closely linked to inflammation, better heart health means less inflammation overall.

Oxidative Stress and Free Radicals

Oxidative stress, which causes inflammation, occurs when there's an imbalance between free radicals and antioxidants in the body. Free radicals are unstable molecules that have an unpaired electron, making them highly reactive. Our body needs them for processes such as energy production in cells and they are used by the immune system to fight infections but we need to keep them in balance.

As an aside, although we are interested in the free radicals made from oxygen here, not all free radicals are made from oxygen (called reactive oxygen species, ROS). Some free radicals can contain different elements like nitrogen, and are called RNS - reactive nitrogen species.

But back to our oxygen-made free radicals. Antioxidants can donate an electron to these free radicals without becoming unstable themselves. This neutralizes them and prevents them from causing harm.

It's when the levels of free radicals become too high and the body doesn't have enough antioxidants to neutralize them, that oxidative stress occurs. It's this which can damage cells, proteins, and DNA, and that contribute to the various health problems, and not only inflammation and heart disease, but cancer as well as 'early' aging.

It goes without saying that to manage oxidative stress, we are aiming to achieve balance between free radicals and antioxidants. Although the body produces some antioxidants naturally, others can be found in foods rich in antioxidants such as fruits, vegetables, nuts, and seeds.

We can also avoid excessive exposure to environmental sources of free radicals such as pollution and tobacco smoke, and adopt a lifestyle that includes regular physical activity and stress management practices like meditation or breathing exercises.

There is also evidence suggesting that certain intermittent fasting methods can help manage oxidative stress. Two popular methods that have been studied are:

Time-Restricted Feeding (TRF): This method includes some of the diets already mentioned and involves eating all meals within a specific window of time each day, typically 8-10 hours, and fasting for the remaining 14-16 hours. Research has shown that TRF can improve metabolic health and autophagy, and reduce oxidative stress markers. (don't worry, this is explained later). A study published in the journal Cell Metabolism found that TRF can lead to significant improvements in oxidative stress and inflammatory markers.

Alternate-Day Fasting (ADF): This method involves alternating between days of normal eating and days of restricted calorie intake (usually around 500-600 calories). Studies have demonstrated that ADF can reduce oxidative stress and improve antioxidant defenses. A study in the journal Free Radical Biology and Medicine found that ADF decreased oxidative stress and enhanced resistance to oxidative damage in both animals and humans.

Both methods involve periods of fasting that stimulate processes like autophagy and mitochondrial function, which helps manage oxidative stress. While more research is needed to fully understand the long-term effects, current evidence supports the idea that intermittent fasting can be an effective strategy for reducing oxidative stress.

Key Takeaways So Far

Intermittent fasting works because it gives the body extended periods without food intake, which allows time for rest and repair. This break from constant digestion and absorption triggers several beneficial processes:

Reduced Inflammation: The body produces fewer pro-inflammatory cytokines and inflammatory markers like CRP.

Improved Insulin Sensitivity: Fasting improves the body's response to insulin, helping to control blood sugar levels and reduce inflammation.

Decreased Visceral Fat: Fasting helps reduce the fat stored around organs, which lowers the production of inflammatory molecules.

Enhanced Autophagy: Fasting improves autophagy, a process where the body cleans out damaged cells and regenerates new ones, improving overall health.

Better Cholesterol Levels: Fasting can lower LDL ("bad" cholesterol) and increase HDL ("good" cholesterol), reducing the risk of heart disease.

Reduced Oxidative Stress: By lowering oxidative stress, fasting helps decrease inflammation and protect against chronic diseases.

Heart Health: Fasting improves heart health by lowering blood pressure and cholesterol levels, further reducing inflammation.

Having looked at the various health benefits of intermittent fasting, including reduced inflammation, improved insulin sensitivity, and touched on autophagy, we will move on to the another important aspect: its effect on metabolic rate - the rate which determines how efficiently our bodies convert food into energy.

Chapter 3

Metabolic Rate & Metabolic Switching

Understanding Metabolic Rate

Before we talk about metabolic switching, we need to understand the basics of metabolic rate and its role in energy balance within the body.

Basal Metabolic Rate (BMR)

At the core of your metabolism is the Basal Metabolic Rate (BMR), which represents the number of calories your body needs to perform essential life-sustaining functions while at rest. These include pumping blood throughout your body, digesting food, breathing, keeping a stable body temperature and growing hair and skin as well as maintaining levels of different chemicals that your body needs. BMR accounts for about 65-75% of your total daily energy use and is influenced by factors such as age, sex, muscle mass, and genetics. Individuals with higher muscle mass tend to have a higher BMR because muscle tissue requires more energy to maintain than fat tissue.

Resting Metabolic Rate (RMR)

You might also hear the term RMR - this measures the amount of energy your body needs to function in the resting state e.g. eating, short walks, using the bathroom, consuming caffeine or tea, and sweating or shivering. We will be talking about BMR.

Thermic Effect of Food (TEF)

Meanwhile, part of your metabolic rate is the Thermic Effect of Food (TEF), which refers to the energy required for digestion and absorption of nutrients. TEF typically accounts for about 10% of your total daily energy use. Different macronutrients (proteins, fats, and carbohydrates) have varying thermic effects, with protein having the highest TEF, meaning it requires more energy to process compared to fats and carbohydrates. It's why a protein-rich diet can burn more energy.

Physical Activity

It won't come as a surprise to learn that physical activity is also a significant part of the metabolic rate. It includes all the calories burned during physical exercise and non-exercise activities such as walking, typing, or even fidgeting! As you would also expect, it can vary greatly from person to person, depending on lifestyle and activity level. I will include a chapter on lifestyle later in the book and provide some exercise examples.

Adaptive Thermogenesis

We also have something called adaptive thermogenesis, which is the body's way of adapting to changes in the environment, such as temperature and diet It represents the energy use beyond the BMR, TEF, and physical activity, and can be influenced by factors like stress and hormonal changes making it of particular interest to women over 50 or those experiencing peri-menopause and beyond and those experiencing menstruation.

Energy Balance

It's pretty obvious that when you consume more calories than your body needs, the excess energy is stored as fat, leading to weight gain while eating fewer calories than needed causes the body to use stored energy, resulting in weight loss.

Metabolic Flexibility

The human body primarily relies on two main energy sources: glucose and fat. When we eat, our bodies typically use glucose from carbohydrates as the main energy source because it is quickly accessible and easy to use. Fat serves as a stored form of energy that the body can use when glucose is not readily available. The ability to switch between these energy sources as needed is known as metabolic flexibility or switching.

Fasting, particularly intermittent fasting, plays a significant role in helping metabolic flexibility. When you fast, the availability of glucose in your bloodstream decreases. From the introduction we know that, initially, the body uses stored glucose, known as glycogen, from the liver and muscles for energy. As glycogen stores become depleted, the body must find an alternative energy source to continue functioning effectively. This is when it begins breaking down stored fat into fatty acids and ketones, the process known as ketosis, which provides an alternative fuel source.

This transition from glucose to ketones and back is what we refer to as metabolic switching. This process is not just about energy - it includes cellular health, impacting our overall well-being. It is also why, if you are over 50, you don't want to fast for more than 36 hours if you don't want to lose muscle mass, or can't afford to and why, before you start any longer fasting regime, you should double check with a doctor or health care provider. It can also impact your hormones.

However, the practice of intermittent fasting trains the body to switch between these energy sources more efficiently. One of the primary benefits is improved insulin sensitivity which helps our cells absorb glucose from the bloodstream. Enhanced insulin sensitivity over time means that the body becomes even more efficient at using glucose when it is available, and the lower insulin levels during fasting periods increases fat burning, helping move the body from using glucose to using the stored fat.

On top of this, regular fasting also improves the body's adaptation to ketosis. Once again, as the body becomes more adept at entering and maintaining this state, it can switch to fat burning more easily (and faster) during extended fasting periods.

One other significant benefit is the improvement of mitochondrial function. Mitochondria play a crucial role in energy production and cellular health. During metabolic switching, your body's energy source shifts from glucose to ketones and fatty acids, removing damaged mitochondria and stimulating the production of new, healthy ones. This process, known as mitophagy, helps reduce oxidative stress and inflammation, once again helping to lower the risk of mutations and cancer. Improved mitochondrial health also supports cellular metabolism and prevents the oxidative stress that contributes to tumor development.

One of the most notable effect of improved metabolic flexibility is better energy levels throughout the day, even when we are not eating regularly. This stable energy is a yet another result of the body's ability to efficiently switch to fat burning during fasting periods. It means that efficient fat burning not only aids in weight management but also improves overall metabolic health.

It is also why, one of the signs of poor metabolic health is feeling constantly tired or lacking energy even after rest or having difficulty recovering from exercise with extended periods of soreness and fatigue after physical activity.

Better metabolic flexibility also contributes to reduced hunger and cravings. As the body becomes more efficient at using fat stores for energy, it can sustain energy levels without constant food intake, leading to greater control over hunger and reduced cravings. This control can be particularly beneficial for helping us stick to a balanced diet and preventing overeating.

Finally, improved physical and mental performance is another key benefit. Metabolic flexibility helps to support physical endurance and mental clarity.

Autophagy & mTOR

One of the most significant benefits of metabolic switching is its role in autophagy - the cellular housekeeping process that takes place when we give our body a break from continuous digestion and absorption. During fasting, autophagy is upregulated, allowing the body to repair itself more efficiently which helps to maintain healthy tissues and organs and, as mentioned, can even play a role in slowing the aging process.

At the same time, fasting stimulates the mammalian target of rapamycin (mTOR) pathway, crucial for cell growth and regeneration including muscle cells. A protein, it helps control how your cells grow, repair and multiply. It also regulates the production of hormones.

While accelerated cell regeneration is a natural response to injury in organs like the liver, to work effectively, it needs to ensure that damaged cells are replaced, not healthy ones and its autophagy that gets rid of the these damaged cells in its clean-up routine.

When you fast, or go without eating for a while, your body takes a break from growing and starts cleaning up and repairing damaged cells. This process is the autophagy part, a recycling system for our cells.

When you start eating again, mTOR gets activated, telling your cells to stop the cleaning process and start growing and building up once more. So, fasting helps make sure your body has time to repair itself (during fasting) and time to grow and build up (during eating). It's this balance which is essential for healthy cellular function and longevity.

Together, these two pathways ensure that the body can efficiently remove toxins, (known as detox pathways) maintain cellular health, and support overall metabolic and physiological balance ie. it can help prevent 'brain fog' - this is helped by BDNF which we talk about shortly.

Excessive and disorganized regeneration, caused by constant mTOR activation from continuous food intake, can lead to accelerated cellular aging, increased risk of mutations, fibrosis, chronic inflammation, and cancers. There are quite a few symptoms of blocked detox pathways that are easy to spot such as chronic fatigue, boating and dry skin or rashes.

It simply means that we need to balance the switching between mTOR and autophagy. We need time to build and grow as well as time to rest and repair, and we can't do both these processes at once.

Ketones and Cancer

Many cancer cells rely heavily on glucose for energy through a process known as aerobic glycolysis or the Warburg effect. Reducing glucose availability through fasting and metabolic switching can potentially starve cancer cells and prevent their growth.

This brings us to Ketones. Ketones provide energy for most organs and are especially important for the brain, which can't directly use fatty acids. As well as this, while cancer cells often struggle to adapt to using ketones for energy, normal cells can switch to ketone metabolism, selectively disadvantaging cancer cells.

Ketosis

There is a point at which fasting prompts the body to switch from using glucose to ketones for energy: a process is known as ketosis.

When you start fasting, your body first uses the glucose available in your bloodstream for energy. After the initial glucose is used up, the body taps into glycogen in the liver and muscles (stored in the form of glucose). This phase can last for about 24-48 hours, depending on your metabolism and activity level.

Once glycogen stores are depleted, the body begins to break down fat into fatty acids and ketones in a process called ketogenesis. Generally, ketosis becomes significant between 24 to 72 hours of continuous fasting.

You can also trigger ketosis by significantly reducing your carbohydrate intake (usually to less than 50 grams per day) and increasing fat intake. This approach, the basis of the Keto Diet, maintains ketosis through macronutrient manipulation, while intermittent fasting focuses on meal timing.

Hormetic Stress

Intermittent fasting also induces a mild form of stress known as hormetic stress. This type of stress makes cells more resilient helping them to become stronger and function more efficiently, much like how muscles grow stronger in response to physical exercise. Essentially hormetic stress improves the body's ability to cope with various stressors.

Symptoms (or problems or solve)

You are probably wondering what the symptoms might be of a low metabolic rate or what general health conditions can be helped by intermittent fasting. These include difficulty sleeping, general tiredness and lack of energy, feelings on anxiety, high blood pressure and difficulty concentrating. These issues can be linked to imbalances in neurotransmitters and hormones.

Role of GABA and BDNF

Sleeplessness and anxiety can be caused by something we have not yet mentioned and its GABA. It's a deficiency or imbalance in GABA that can contribute to sleeplessness and anxiety. GABA is a neurotransmitter that helps to reduce neuronal excitability leading to reduced stress and anxiety levels, and there is evidence that fasting improves GABA levels.

Fasting also helps increase levels of Brain-Derived Neurotrophic Factor (BDNF), which supports the growth, differentiation, and survival of neurons. Higher levels of BDNF are linked to improved learning, memory, and cognitive function and may protect against neurodegenerative diseases like Alzheimer's and Parkinson's.

Managing Autoimmune Conditions

The effects of metabolic switching extend to autoimmune conditions by repairing the gut and mitochondria and regulating gene expression. Fasting can help manage and potentially improve autoimmune issues by promoting healthier cellular function.

Intermittent Fasting

The 16:8 intermittent fasting method, where you fast for 16 hours and eat during an 8-hour window, can still be effective for weight loss, even though it might not push the body into a deep state of ketosis as longer fasts do. In fact, even the 12:12 can have an effect.

Fasting for 12, 14 or 16 hours can improve insulin sensitivity and reduce insulin levels, helping the body burn fat more efficiently and it can also influence hunger and satiety hormones, such as ghrelin and leptin, reducing overeating.

Even without reaching deep ketosis, intermittent fasting can improve metabolic health, including better lipid profiles and reduced inflammation.

Importantly, many people find it more sustainable and easier to stick to compared to longer fasting periods or strict diets like Keto.

Excessive Fasting

I will mentioned excessive fasting at this point and before we move on to the information we need on food, energy and the fasting methods that are easy to do.

Excessive fasting generally refers to fasting periods that are too long or too frequent and it isn't good for you.

Inadequate caloric intake can result in significant weight loss, muscle wasting, fatigue, and compromised immune function while too frequent fasting with very short eating windows may not allow the body enough time to recover and receive the nutrition it needs. If you are considering any type of dramatic fasting then you really should talk to a health care professional to ensure you are giving your body what it needs.

Here are a few examples:

Fasting for Too Many Consecutive Days: Extended fasting periods lasting several days without medical supervision can be potentially harmful. For example, fasting for more than 3-5 consecutive days without proper nutrition and hydration can lead to nutrient deficiencies, muscle loss, and other health issues.

Inadequate Caloric Intake: Regularly fasting in a way that leads to consistently low caloric intake can result in significant weight loss, muscle wasting, fatigue, and compromised immune function.

Too Frequent Fasting: Fasting with very short eating windows and minimal rest periods between fasting cycles can be excessive. For instance, continuously practicing 20-hour fasts with only a 4-hour eating window every day may not allow the body enough time to recover and receive the nutrition it needs.

Ignoring Body Signals: If fasting leads to persistent feelings of extreme hunger, dizziness, fatigue, or other signs of physical distress, it may be excessive. Ignoring these signals can result in long-term harm.

Impact on Metabolic Health: Excessive fasting can slow down metabolism if the body perceives it as prolonged starvation. This can lead to a decrease in metabolic rate and adverse effects on thyroid function and overall energy balance.

Medical Conditions: Individuals with certain medical conditions, such as diabetes, eating disorders, or severe nutritional deficiencies, should always check with a health professional.

It all means that it is important to approach fasting with balance.

Signs of Poor or Weak Metabolic Health

Obvious signs of poor metabolic health can manifest in various ways throughout the body. Here are some key indicators. Start keeping a track of how you are feeling to get an idea of your metabolic health by using the tracker at the end of this chapter.

1. Weight Gain and Obesity
Unexplained Weight Gain: Gaining weight despite no significant changes in diet or exercise.
Central Obesity: Accumulation of fat around the abdomen, leading to an "apple-shaped" body.

2. Fatigue and Low Energy
Chronic Fatigue: Feeling constantly tired or lacking energy even after adequate rest.
Difficulty Recovering from Exercise: Extended periods of soreness and fatigue after physical activity.

3. Digestive Issues
Bloating and Gas: Persistent bloating and excessive gas.
Constipation or Diarrhea: Irregular bowel movements and digestive discomfort.

4. Skin Problems
Acne and Rashes: Frequent skin breakouts and rashes.
Dark Patches on Skin: Areas of darkened skin, especially around the neck and armpits (acanthosis nigricans), which can indicate insulin resistance.

5. Hormonal Imbalances
Irregular Menstrual Cycles: Disrupted or irregular periods in women.
Decreased Libido: Reduced interest in sexual activity.

6. Cardiovascular Symptoms
High Blood Pressure: Consistently elevated blood pressure readings.
High Cholesterol Levels: Elevated levels of LDL (bad) cholesterol and triglycerides, along with low levels of HDL (good) cholesterol.

7. Blood Sugar Issues
High Blood Sugar Levels: Elevated fasting blood glucose levels or abnormal results in glucose tolerance tests.
Frequent Urination and Thirst: Signs of high blood sugar levels, often seen in diabetes.

8. Mental and Cognitive Issues
Brain Fog: Difficulty concentrating, memory problems, and general mental sluggishness.
Mood Swings and Irritability: Increased sensitivity and frequent mood changes.

9. Sleep Problems
Poor Sleep Quality: Trouble falling asleep, staying asleep, or waking up feeling unrefreshed.
Sleep Apnea: Pauses in breathing during sleep, often associated with obesity.

10. Poor Immune Function
Frequent Infections: Increased susceptibility to colds, flu, and other infections.
Slow Healing: Delayed healing of wounds and infections.

11. Inflammation and Pain
Joint and Muscle Pain: Unexplained aches, pains, and stiffness.
Chronic Inflammation: Persistent low-grade inflammation, often detectable through markers like C-reactive protein (CRP).

12. Metabolic Syndrome Indicators

Waist Circumference: Waist circumference (over 40 inches)
High Blood Pressure: Readings consistently above 130/85 mmHg.
High Blood Sugar: Fasting glucose levels above 100 mg/dL.
High Triglycerides: Levels above 150 mg/dL.
Low HDL Cholesterol: Below 40 mg/dL for men and 50 mg/dL for women

Tips and Tools

Today, estimating your metabolic rate is easier than ever with the availability of bathroom scales that include apps to measure your BMR, typically starting at around £20 (or $25).

Managing stress and maintaining healthy cortisol levels is always good for you for many reasons.

For immediate stress relief, try breathing in through your nose for a count of 4, holding for a count of 7, then breath and out through your mouth for a count of 8 and repeat at least 4 or 5 times.

Before you begin deeply exhale through your mouth (purse your lips to make whooshing sound), then during the exercise, try to keep your tongue positioned toward the roof of the mouth, with the tip of your tongue touching the back of your front teeth.

Chapter 4

Exercises

Quiz

1. What is metabolic switching and what are the two primary energy sources the body uses in this process?

A) Transition between sleep and wakefulness using proteins and carbohydrates.
B) Transition between using glucose and ketones for energy.
C) Switching between different types of diets to avoid food allergies.
D) Changing exercise routines to boost metabolism.

2. Why is constant availability and consumption of food problematic for metabolic health?

A) It leads to a decrease in energy levels.
B) It prevents the body from entering a state of ketosis and autophagy.
C) It causes the body to use only proteins for energy.
D) It increases the body's reliance on glucose only.

3. What cellular process does fasting activate that helps clean up damaged components within cells?

A) mTOR pathway.
B) Autophagy.
C) Glycolysis.
D) Lipolysis

4. Which of the following is NOT a benefit of metabolic switching mentioned in the text?

A) Slows down the aging process.
B) Increases dependence on medication.
C) Mobilizes toxins.
D) Powers up memory.

5. How often do liver cells completely replace themselves?

A) Every 5 days.
B) Every 2 to 4 weeks.
C) 150 to 500 days.
D) Every 7 years.

6. What is the role of mTOR in the body?

A) It is responsible for cell death and clearance.
B) It is a cellular growth pathway that supports hormone production and muscle growth.
C) It breaks down fat for energy.
D) It reduces the body's ability to adapt to stress.

7. What are the signs that may indicate your body's detox pathways are congested?

A) Increased energy levels.
B) Rashes and brain fog.
C) Reduced appetite.
D) Improved sleep quality.

8. How can metabolic switching impact cancer?

A) By permanently eliminating cancer cells.
B) By enhancing mitochondrial function, which can prevent dysfunctional cells from developing into cancer.
C) By increasing mTOR activity to fight cancer cells.
D) By stopping the production of ATP in cells.

9. What hormone-like substance increases in the brain during fasting and contributes to neuron growth?

A) Insulin.
B) Cortisol.
C) Brain-derived neurotrophic factor (BDNF).
D) Adrenaline.

Quiz Answers

1. B - Transition between using glucose and ketones for energy.
2. B - It prevents the body from entering a state of ketosis and autophagy.
3. B - Autophagy.
4. B - Increases dependence on medication.
5. C - 150 to 500 days.
6. B - It is a cellular growth pathway that supports hormone production and muscle growth.
7. B - Rashes and brain fog.
8. B - By enhancing mitochondrial function, which can prevent dysfunctional cells from developing into cancer.
9. C - Brain-derived neurotrophic factor (BDNF).

Exercises

Document your current eating patterns, including the number of meals you have per day and the typical length of your overnight fast. This baseline information will help you understand your starting point before implementing metabolic switching.

Mitochondrial health is central to the chapter's teaching, Note any symptoms (such as chronic fatigue or muscle weakness) and include your energy levels, cognitive function, digestive health, or any symptoms that might indicate poor metabolic health (like fatigue post-meals). Refer to this at a later date to track any improvements.

Metabolic Switching Symptom Tracker

The following is an example of a Metabolic Switching Symptom Tracker:

It includes a daily log over 2 pages, then a weekly summary and reflection.

This is also included at the end of this workbook and covers a period of a month. You might want to fill out this tracker to get into the habit of noting what and when you eat, and how you feel.

Notes

Energy Levels: How energetic do you feel? Are you able to complete your daily activities with ease?

Mental Clarity: How clear is your thinking? Can you focus and remember things well?

Digestive Health: How is your digestion? Any discomfort, bloating, or irregularities?

Mood: How do you feel emotionally? Any changes in your mood or stress levels?

Physical Activity: What type and how much physical activity did you do?

Sleep Quality: How many hours did you sleep and how restful was it?

Overall Well-Being: Considering all factors, how do you rate your overall feeling of health and wellness?

Exercises

Instructions

Fill in the tracker daily, ideally at the same time each day for consistency.

Rate your energy levels, mental clarity, digestive health, mood, and overall well-being on a scale of 1 to 10, with 1 being very poor and 10 being excellent.

Use the weekly reflection to summarize your observations and note any trends or significant changes.

Begin by noting the following:

Personal Information

Current Weight:

Height:

Age:

Date	Energy Level (1-10)	Mental Clarity (1-10)	Digestive Health (1-10)	Digestive Health (1-10)	Mood (1-10)	Physical Acitivty (1-10)	Sleep Quality incl Hrs (1-10)	Unusual Symptoms	Overall Well-being (1-10)

Instructions:
- Rate your energy levels, mental clarity, digestive health, mood, and overall well-being on a scale of 1 to 10.
- Note the type and duration of physical activity.
- Record sleep duration and quality, along with any unusual symptoms you might experience.

Date	Energy Level (1-10)	Mental Clarity (1-10)	Digestive Health (1-10)	Digestive Health (1-10)	Mood (1-10)	Physical Acitivty (1-10)	Sleep Quality incl Hrs (1-10)	Unusual Symptoms	Overall Well-being (1-10)

Instructions:
- Rate your energy levels, mental clarity, digestive health, mood, and overall well-being on a scale of 1 to 10.
- Note the type and duration of physical activity.
- Record sleep duration and quality, along with any unusual symptoms you might experience.

Chapter 5

What Not To Eat

Now would be a good time to take a look at what not to eat, and which foods look like they are diet-friendly, but might not be very good for you (if you were calorie counting only).

Today's rise in obesity and type 2 diabetes has gone hand-in-hand with dietary trends that promote low-fat, high-sugar foods and processed foods. According the Cleveland Clinic, these processed foods can lead to insulin resistance, where your cells struggle to use insulin properly, causing energy depletion and fat storage. This is a precursor to type 2 diabetes and other metabolic issues. We cover some of these as part of explaining the glycemic load as well as

Chronic stress also plays a role by increasing cortisol levels, which raises glucose levels and alters insulin response. This disruption in metabolic health makes weight loss and overall well-being more challenging. For women, 'Obesogens'—chemicals found in food and the environment—can disrupt hormonal functions, leading to weight gain and other health issues. And they can effect men too. These chemicals are often found in processed foods, plastics, and other everyday products and we have listed some below.

Hormonal fluctuations during menstrual cycles, pregnancy, or menopause can also impact how our bodies respond to diets. This is why personalising your diet to meet your hormonal changes can help address related issues. We will cover these in a later chapter, and before we move on, let's take a look at what not to eat.

Next, we'll explore what to use and what to avoid as we start to evaluate our current habits and make positive changes. At the end of this section there are worksheets for you to complete that will get you thinking about what you are eating.

Foods Low in Calories but Also Low in Nutrients

While many people aim to include low-calorie foods in their diets to manage weight, it's essential to ensure that these foods also provide necessary nutrients. Here are some examples of low-calorie foods that are often low in nutrients, which might be mistakenly considered healthy diet options:

Rice Cakes

- **Nutrient Profile**: Mostly carbohydrates with very little fiber, protein, vitamins, or minerals.
- **Why Misleading**: Often considered a healthy snack due to low calories, but they provide minimal nutritional value and can lead to spikes in blood sugar.

Diet Sodas

- **Nutrient Profile**: Virtually no calories, vitamins, or minerals.
- **Why Misleading**: Seen as a calorie-free alternative to sugary drinks, but they offer no nutritional benefits and may contain artificial sweeteners.

Light or Fat-Free Salad Dressings

- **Nutrient Profile**: Low in calories and fats but often high in sugar and lacking essential vitamins.
- **Why Misleading**: Chosen to reduce calorie intake, yet they often have added sugars and lack the healthy fats needed to absorb fat-soluble vitamins in salads.

Cucumber

- **Nutrient Profile**: Very low in calories and mostly water, with small amounts of vitamins and minerals.
- **Why Misleading**: While hydrating and refreshing, cucumbers offer minimal nutritional value compared to other vegetables.

Celery

- **Nutrient Profile**: Low in calories and fiber, with minimal vitamins and minerals.
- **Why Misleading**: Often touted as a negative-calorie food, it doesn't provide much in terms of essential nutrients.

Sugar-Free Gelatin Desserts

- **Nutrient Profile**: Low in calories, high in artificial colors and sweeteners, with no vitamins or minerals.
- **Why Misleading**: Marketed as a guilt-free dessert, these offer no nutritional value and contain artificial additives.

Air-Popped Popcorn

- **Nutrient Profile**: Low in calories and fiber, but lacks significant amounts of protein, vitamins, or minerals.

- **Why Misleading**: While it can be a low-calorie snack, it is not nutrient-dense unless fortified or eaten with added nutritional toppings.

Sugar-Free Candy

- **Nutrient Profile**: Low in calories and sugar, but also devoid of any vitamins or minerals and often contains artificial ingredients.
- **Why Misleading**: Chosen as a low-calorie sweet treat, it provides no nutritional value and can lead to digestive issues due to sugar alcohols.

100-Calorie Snack Packs

- **Nutrient Profile**: Low in calories but typically high in refined carbohydrates and lacking fiber, protein, vitamins, and minerals.
- **Why Misleading**: Seen as a portion-controlled snack option, but they often contain processed ingredients and lack essential nutrients.

Flavored Water

- **Nutrient Profile**: Low in calories but often contains artificial flavors and sweeteners without any vitamins or minerals.
- **Why Misleading**: Marketed as a healthy hydration option, but it can contain additives.

There is nothing wrong with including these foods in a balanced diet, but they should not be relied upon as primary sources of nutrition.

Common Obesogens and Their Sources

Obesogens are chemicals that can disrupt the endocrine system and potentially contribute to weight gain and obesity. They tend to impact women more than men because the endocrine system, which produces hormones such as estrogen and progesterone, is more heavily involved in women's physiology. These chemicals can interfere with the body's metabolism, fat storage, and appetite regulation.

The impact of obesogens can vary before and after menopause due to differences in hormonal levels and the way the endocrine system functions during these periods.

Before Menopause

Before menopause, women experience regular fluctuations in hormones such as estrogen and progesterone as part of their menstrual cycle. The endocrine system is actively producing these hormones in varying amounts throughout the cycle, which could potentially make the body more susceptible to disruptions caused by obesogens. The hormonal fluctuations might amplify the effects of obesogens on metabolism, fat storage, and appetite regulation, possibly contributing to weight gain.

After Menopause

After menopause, the production of estrogen and progesterone decreases significantly, and the hormonal fluctuations become less pronounced. While this might reduce the direct hormonal disruptions caused by obesogens, the changes in body composition, such as increased visceral fat and decreased muscle mass, could still make women vulnerable to the metabolic effects of obesogens. Additionally, postmenopausal women often experience a natural decline in metabolic rate, which could exacerbate the impact of obesogens on weight gain and fat storage.

While obesogens can have significant effects both before and after menopause, their impact might differ due to the changes in hormonal levels and metabolism. Before menopause, the endocrine system's active hormone production could make women more susceptible to obesogen disruptions. After menopause, the decreased hormonal fluctuations and changes in body composition might still leave women vulnerable to the effects of these chemicals, albeit in different ways.

Although the impact of obesogens might be more pronounced in women due to their hormonal fluctuations and the significant role of estrogen and progesterone, men are also susceptible to the effects of these chemicals. In men, obesogens can disrupt metabolism, increase fat storage, affect appetite regulation, and lead to a range of health issues, including metabolic syndrome, reduced muscle mass, and insulin resistance.

We list the most common with their side effects below before giving examples of where you might find them. These chemicals are found in various foods, packaging materials, and household products.

Bisphenol A (BPA)

- **Sources**: Plastics, canned food linings, thermal paper receipts.
- **Health Effects**: BPA is known to disrupt endocrine function by mimicking estrogen, which can lead to hormonal imbalances. In men, BPA exposure has been linked to decreased testosterone levels. Linked to increased fat accumulation and obesity, insulin resistance, and an increased risk of developing type 2 diabetes.

Phthalates

- **Sources**: Plastics, personal care products, food packaging.

- **Health Effects**: Interfere with hormone function, linked to weight gain and insulin resistance.
- Phthalates can interfere with the production and function of testosterone, leading to reduced sperm quality and lower testosterone levels.

Perfluorinated Chemicals (PFCs) and Perfluorooctanoic Acid (PFOA)

- **Sources**: Non-stick cookware, stain-resistant fabrics, food packaging
- **Health Effects**: Associated with disruptions in lipid metabolism, leading to increased cholesterol levels and changes in body fat distribution. Studies have shown that PFOA can interfere with hormone regulation and contribute to obesity, iver damage, and metabolic syndrome.

Atrazine

- **Sources**: Herbicides used on crops.
- **Health Effects**: Associated with increased fat storage and endocrine disruption.

Organotins

- **Sources**: Pesticides, antifouling paints, PVC plastics.
- **Health Effects**: Linked to increased fat cell production and obesity.

Polychlorinated Biphenyls (PCBs)

Sources: Industrial products, contaminated food and water.

Health Effects: Disrupt endocrine function, linked to weight gain and metabolic disorders.

Tributyltin (TBT)

Sources: TBT is an organotin compound used in marine antifouling paints, industrial water systems, and as a biocide in various products.

Impact: TBT has been shown to activate receptors that regulate fat cell production and storage, leading to increased fat accumulation. In animal studies, TBT exposure has resulted in obesity, insulin resistance, and liver steatosis (fatty liver disease). The effects in humans are still being studied, but the potential for significant metabolic disruption makes TBT a concern.

Dichlorodiphenyltrichloroethane (DDT)

- **Sources**: Pesticides (now banned but still present in the environment).

- **Health Effects**: Linked to obesity and diabetes.

Identifying Exposure Obesogens

To determine if obesogens are present in your food cupboard, (or home) check for the following:

Packaging: The goal here is to avoid exposure to harmful chemicals like BPA and phthalates. Look for plastic containers that are labeled BPA-free. Avoid plastics with recycling codes 3 (phthalates) and 7 (often indicates BPA). A Chinese doctor friend told me to remove all plastic food packaging from fruit and veg as soon as I get home, and immediately wash the food. He maintains that the chemicals found it food wrapping seeps into the food and removing the plastic exposure as soon as possible is always the best course of action.

Canned Foods: Traditional canned foods often have linings that contain BPA so choose canned foods that are labeled as BPA-free.

Processed Foods: Highly processed foods may contain various additives and chemicals. Check ingredient lists for unfamiliar additives and avoid those with long lists of synthetic ingredients.

Non-Stick Cookware: Avoid using old or scratched non-stick cookware that may release PFCs. It's very difficult to know what your non-stick pans are made of (I know, I have tried). Most modern ones are safe, but older ones not so much. If you are using old pans just make sure they are not scratched because, if they do contain PFCs the scratches will help to release them into your food.

Produce: Choose organic produce to reduce exposure to pesticides like atrazine and organotins. You might want to consider frozen vegetables if you can't source organic. Frozen vegetables are typically blanched (briefly cooked) before freezing and this process can reduce pesticide residues. Additionally, frozen vegetables are often harvested at peak ripeness and immediately processed, potentially reducing their exposure to pesticides that would otherwise be used during storage and transportation. As always, it is still important to check the labelling,

Personal Care Products: Check labels for phthalates and avoid products with "fragrance" listed as an ingredient, as it can be a source of phthalates.

Synthetic Ingredients Found in Common Foods

Artificial Sweeteners

- **Aspartame**: Found in diet sodas, sugar-free gum, and low-calorie desserts.
- **Sucralose**: Used in sugar-free baked goods, beverages, and candies.
- **Saccharin**: Present in diet sodas, sugar-free chewing gum, and sweetener packets.

Preservatives

- **Sodium Benzoate**: Common in soft drinks, salad dressings, and condiments.
- **Potassium Sorbate**: Found in cheese, wine, yogurt, and baked goods.
- **BHA/BHT** (Butylated Hydroxyanisole/Butylated Hydroxytoluene): Used in snack foods, cereals, and processed meats.

Artificial Colors

- **Red 40 (Allura Red)**: Present in candies, baked goods, and cereals.
- **Yellow 5 (Tartrazine)**: Found in sodas, chips, and candies.
- **Blue 1 (Brilliant Blue)**: Used in beverages, candies, and ice creams.

Flavor Enhancers

- **Monosodium Glutamate (MSG)**: Common in savory snacks, soups, and Chinese food.
- **Disodium Inosinate and Disodium Guanylate**: Often found in instant noodles, chips, and processed meats.

Emulsifiers and Stabilizers

- **Lecithin**: Used in chocolate, margarine, and salad dressings.
- **Polysorbate 80**: Found in ice cream, salad dressings, and sauces.
- **Carboxymethyl Cellulose (CMC)**: Present in baked goods, ice cream, and dairy products.

Artificial Flavors

Vanillin: Used as a vanilla flavoring in ice cream, baked goods, and candies.

Ethyl Maltol: Provides a sweet, caramel-like flavor in candies, baked goods, and beverages.

Texturizers

- **Modified Food Starch**: Used in soups, sauces, and frozen meals.
- **Xanthan Gum**: Found in salad dressings, sauces, and gluten-free baked goods.
- **Carrageenan**: Present in dairy products, plant-based milk, and deli meats.

Sweeteners

- **High Fructose Corn Syrup (HFCS)**: Common in sodas, candies, baked goods, and breakfast cereals.

Anti-Caking Agents

- **Silicon Dioxide**: Used in powdered foods like spices, coffee creamer, and soup mixes.
- **Calcium Silicate**: Found in salt, baking powder, and dry mixes.

Gelling Agents

- **Agar-Agar**: Used in jellies, desserts, and dairy products.
- **Pectin**: Common in jams, jellies, and yogurts.

Actions to minimise exposure to Obesogens

- **Choose Fresh, Whole Foods**: Prioritize fresh, whole foods over processed and packaged foods.
- **Use Glass or Stainless Steel**: Store food in glass or stainless steel containers instead of plastic.
- **Filter Drinking Water**: Use a water filter to reduce contaminants like PFCs and PCBs.
- **Avoid Non-Stick Cookware**: Use alternatives like cast iron or stainless steel cookware or check that your cookware is not scratched and not made of the older non-stick formula that contains obesogens.
- **Opt for Organic**: When possible, choose organic fruits, vegetables, and meats to reduce pesticide exposure.
- **Check Labels**: Read labels on food and personal care products to avoid harmful chemicals.

- **Ventilate Your Home**: Ensure good ventilation to reduce indoor air pollutants.

Foods to Avoid

Bad Oils

These include partially hydrogenated oils, corn oil, cottonseed oil, canola oil, vegetable oil, soybean oil, safflower oil, and sunflower oil. These oils are known to cause cellular inflammation and contribute to insulin resistance. They are often hidden in processed foods and can exacerbate hunger and cravings.

Refined Sugars and Flours

High on the glycemic index, these include breads, pastas, crackers, and desserts. They can lead to blood sugar spikes and crashes, fueling a cycle of cravings and overeating. These foods are also linked to inflammation and can disrupt metabolic health.

Chemical Additives

We have covered some of these in detail above but as a rule of thumb avoid artificial colors, flavorings, red or blue dyes, saccharin, Nutra-Sweet, and Splenda are examples. These synthetic ingredients can contribute to insulin resistance - there are obesogens, meaning they can disrupt hormonal balance and lead to weight gain.

Chapter 6

Glycemic Load Matters

Foods affect blood sugar levels differently, and understanding the glycemic index is key to managing this.

The Glycemic Index (GI) is a ranking system that measures how quickly a carbohydrate-containing food raises blood glucose levels after consumption. Foods are scored on a scale from 0 to 100, with higher values indicating that the food causes a more rapid increase in blood glucose levels.

Foods with a low glycemic index, like avocados, are preferable because they do not spike blood sugar and insulin levels, helping to maintain energy balance and support metabolic health. In fact, avocados have a very low GI, typically around 15. This makes them an excellent choice for a low-GI diet. Avocados have the added benefit of not only low in carbohydrates, but they are also rich in healthy fats, fiber, vitamins, and minerals.

Although low GI is great, it's okay to eat those foods with medium GI, and even sometimes foods with a high GI index. But its always good to know if you are! As always, the mix is about balance and there are some examples in this chapter.

Categories of Glycemic Index

Low GI Foods (55 or less)

These foods cause a slow, gradual rise in blood glucose levels.

Here are some examples of low-GI foods:

Fruits and Vegetables

- Avocados
- Berries: Blueberries, strawberries, raspberries, and blackberries
- Cherries
- Plums
- Grapefruit
- Pears
- Apples
- Oranges
- Peaches
- Leafy Greens: Spinach, kale, and Swiss chard
- Broccoli
- Cauliflower
- Carrots
- Tomatoes
- Zucchini
- Bell Peppers
- Eggplant

Whole Grains

- Steel-cut oats
- Rolled oats
- Quinoa
- Barley
- Brown rice
- Bulgur
- Whole grain pasta

Legumes

- Lentils
- Chickpeas
- Kidney beans
- Black beans
- Navy beans
- Peas

Dairy and Alternatives

- Milk (full-fat or skim)
- Yogurt (especially Greek yogurt)
- Cheese
- Soy milk

Nuts and Seeds

- Almonds
- Walnuts
- Chia seeds
- Flaxseeds
- Pumpkin seeds

Proteins

- Lean meats: Chicken, turkey, and lean cuts of beef and pork
- Fish: Salmon, mackerel, and sardines
- Eggs
- Tofu
- Tempeh

Breads and Cereals

- Whole grain bread
- Sourdough bread
- Pumpernickel bread
- Bran cereal

Snacks

- Hummus with vegetable sticks
- Nut butter on whole grain toast
- Greek yogurt with a handful of berries
- Cottage cheese with sliced vegetables

Medium GI Foods (56-69)

These foods cause a moderate increase in blood glucose levels which means that they can provide a balanced source of energy without causing the rapid blood sugar spikes associated with high-GI foods. You can combine medium-GI foods with low-GI foods to help maintain a more stable blood sugar levels throughout the day too.

Grains and Cereals

- Whole Wheat Bread: GI around 69
- Pita Bread: GI around 57-68
- Quick Oats: GI around 65
- Muesli: GI around 57-69
- Couscous: GI around 65

Rice and Pasta

- Basmati Rice: GI around 58-65
- Brown Rice: GI around 68
- Whole Grain Pasta: GI around 55-68

Fruits

- Bananas: GI around 56-62 (depending on ripeness)
- Mangoes: GI around 56-60
- Papayas: GI around 56-60
- Raisins: GI around 64

Starchy Vegetables

- Sweet Corn: GI around 60
- Yams: GI around 61
- New Potatoes: GI around 62

Dairy and Alternatives

- Ice Cream: GI around 57-65 (depending on sugar and fat content)
- Custard: GI around 58

Snacks

- Popcorn (air-popped, no added sugar): GI around 55-65
- Digestive Biscuits: GI around 63

Sugary Foods and Sweets

- Sucrose (table sugar): GI around 65
- Jams and Marmalades: GI around 55-65 (depending on sugar content)

Beverages

- Orange Juice: GI around 56-66
- Soft Drinks: GI around 59-65 (depending on sugar content)

High GI Foods (70 and above)

Foods with a glycemic index (GI) of 70 or above are considered high-GI foods.

High GI foods are quickly broken down and absorbed into the bloodstream, leading to a rapid increase in blood glucose levels which causes a sharp spike in blood sugar shortly after eating.

The rapid rise in blood glucose levels triggers a corresponding spike in insulin release from the pancreas. If you eat a lot of foods with a high GI, the frequent spikes in insulin levels can lead to insulin resistance, and this is a significant risk factor for developing type 2 diabetes. It means that managing blood glucose levels through diet can help prevent this condition.

To make matters worse, the quick spike in blood sugar is often followed by a rapid decline, leading to what we know as a "sugar crash." It is this what causes feelings of hunger and fatigue shortly after eating, which can result in overeating and poor energy levels.

High GI foods can also contribute to weight gain through increased fat storage, especially around the abdominal area. This is not helped by the rapid increase and subsequent crash in blood sugar levels which that can lead to overeating that we just mentioned.

It all means that insulin resistance and obesity can be the result of a diet high in high GI foods. On top of this, they are also risk factors for cardiovascular diseases.

Here are some examples of high-GI foods:

Grains and Cereals

- White Bread: GI around 70-75
- Bagels: GI around 70-75
- Cornflakes: GI around 81-83

- Rice Krispies: GI around 82
- Instant Oatmeal: GI around 79

Rice and Pasta

- White Rice: GI around 72-89 (depending on the type and cooking method)
- Rice Pasta: GI around 92

Snacks

- Pretzels: GI around 83
- Rice Cakes: GI around 82-91
- Popcorn: GI around 72

Fruits and Vegetables

- Watermelon: GI around 72
- Pineapple: GI around 70
- Baked Potatoes: GI around 85
- French Fries: GI around 75-85
- Pumpkin: GI around 75

Sugary Foods and Sweets

- Glucose (Dextrose): GI of 100
- Honey: GI around 58-85 (depending on type)
- Jelly Beans: GI around 78-80
- Doughnuts: GI around 75

Processed Foods

- Instant Noodles: GI around 70-75
- Processed Breakfast Bars: GI around 70-75

Drinks

- Sports Drinks: GI around 78
- Cola: GI around 70

Tips for Managing Glycemic Index

- Choose Low to Medium GI Foods by opting for whole grains, legumes, fruits, and vegetables that have a lower GI. They provide a more sustained release of energy and help maintain stable blood glucose levels.
- Combining high GI foods with low GI foods can help balance the overall glycemic load of a meal. For example, pairing white rice with beans or adding vegetables to a pasta dish can slow down the absorption of glucose.
- High-fiber foods tend to have a lower GI and can help slow the absorption of glucose.
- Include plenty of vegetables, fruits, whole grains, and legumes in your diet.
- Adding healthy fats and proteins to meals can also slow down the absorption of carbohydrates and lower the glycemic impact. Examples include nuts, seeds, avocado, and lean meats.

Planning an intermittent fasting diet with GI and nutrients

You now need to have an idea of what can be added to what, and when a medium (or even high) GI might be okay.

As you begin to plan your intermittent fasting diet, it's important to consider the nutrient content of your foods, and consider their glycemic index (GI), and their level of macronutrients (carbohydrates, proteins, fats), fiber, vitamins, and minerals.

We will cover more on nutrients, proteins and vitamins in the next chapter, but here is an overview of the nutritional content of the medium-GI foods listed, which we categorized as low, medium, or high in terms of overall nutrient quality. It a useful way to get a quick idea of what you might want to work with.

Grains and Cereals

Whole Wheat Bread:

- **Nutrient Content**: Medium to high (fiber, B vitamins, iron)
- **Considerations**: Provides essential nutrients but watch portion size to avoid excess carbs.

Pita Bread:

- **Nutrient Content**: Medium (fiber, protein, some B vitamins)
- **Considerations**: Whole grain versions are preferable for added nutrients.

Quick Oats:

- **Nutrient Content**: Medium (fiber, iron, B vitamins)
- **Considerations**: Good source of fiber and energy; combine with protein or fat to balance.

Muesli:

- **Nutrient Content**: Medium to high (fiber, protein, healthy fats, vitamins, minerals)
- **Considerations**: Choose varieties with minimal added sugar.

Couscous:

- **Nutrient Content**: Medium (protein, selenium)
- **Considerations**: Pair with vegetables and protein for a balanced meal.

Rice and Pasta

Basmati Rice:

- **Nutrient Content**: Medium (some vitamins and minerals, lower fiber)
- **Considerations**: Choose brown basmati for more fiber.

Brown Rice:

- **Nutrient Content**: High (fiber, magnesium, B vitamins)
- **Considerations**: Nutrient-dense, good for IF; watch portion size for carb intake.

Whole Grain Pasta:

- **Nutrient Content**: Medium to high (fiber, protein, B vitamins)
- **Considerations**: More nutrient-dense than refined pasta; pair with vegetables and protein.

Fruits and Vegetables

Bananas:

- **Nutrient Content**: Medium (potassium, vitamin C, vitamin B6, fiber)
- **Considerations**: Good for energy; eat with protein or fat to slow sugar absorption.

Mangoes:

- **Nutrient Content**: High (vitamin C, vitamin A, fiber)
- **Considerations**: Nutrient-rich but higher in natural sugars; moderate portion size.

Papayas:

- **Nutrient Content**: High (vitamin C, vitamin A, folate, fiber)
- **Considerations**: Nutrient-dense; beneficial for digestion.

Raisins:

- **Nutrient Content**: Medium (iron, potassium, fiber, antioxidants)
- **Considerations**: High in natural sugars; use in small amounts

Sweet Corn:

Nutrient Content: Medium (fiber, vitamins B and C, magnesium)

Considerations: Good source of fiber and essential nutrients.

Yams:

Nutrient Content: High (fiber, potassium, vitamin C, vitamin B6)

Considerations: Nutrient-dense; better option than white potatoes.

New Potatoes:

Nutrient Content: Medium (vitamin C, potassium, fiber if skin is consumed)

Considerations: Opt for boiled or baked to maintain nutrients.

Dairy and Alternatives

Ice Cream:

- **Nutrient Content**: Low to medium (calcium, protein, but high in sugars and fats)
- **Considerations**: Treat as an occasional indulgence due to high sugar content.

Custard:

- **Nutrient Content**: Medium (calcium, vitamin D, protein, but high in sugars)
- **Considerations**: Similar to ice cream; moderate consumption.

Snacks

Popcorn (air-popped, no added sugar):

- **Nutrient Content**: Medium (fiber, antioxidants)
- **Considerations**: Healthy snack if not overloaded with butter or salt.

Digestive Biscuits:

- **Nutrient Content**: Low to medium (fiber, but can be high in sugar and fats)
- **Considerations**: Choose whole grain varieties and consume in moderation.

Sugary Foods and Sweets

Sucrose (table sugar):

- **Nutrient Content**: Low (empty calories)
- **Considerations**: Use sparingly.

Jams and Marmalades:

- **Nutrient Content:** Low to medium (vitamins from fruit, but high in sugar)
- **Considerations:** Opt for low-sugar versions.

Beverages

Orange Juice:

- **Nutrient Content:** Medium to high (vitamin C, potassium, folate, but high in sugar)
- **Considerations:** Choose whole fruit over juice for fiber benefits.

Soft Drinks:

- **Nutrient Content:** Low (high in sugar, empty calories)
- **Considerations:** Best to avoid or limit intake.

Overall, you are aiming to incorporate a variety of nutrient-dense foods, particularly those with a medium GI, to maintain balanced blood sugar levels and provide essential nutrients.

Prioritize whole grains, fruits, vegetables, and lean proteins, and be mindful of portion sizes and the overall nutritional profile of your meals. Combining foods with different GIs can help achieve a more balanced nutrient intake and stable energy levels throughout the fasting and eating periods.

Chapter 7

Foods to Eat

Before we take a look at a what 'should' be in your cupboard we are going to bring together inflammation, metabolic rate and the role of intermittent fasting and summarise what we have learned so far in relation to our food.

To do so, it is useful to understand what cofactors are.

In the context of cellular health and nutrient needs, a cofactor refers to a non-protein chemical compound or metallic ion that is required for an enzyme's activity as a catalyst. ie. if helps make it react (and if often needed for any reaction to take place).

Role of Cofactors in Cellular Functions

Energy Production

Magnesium acts as a cofactor in many ATP-generating reactions. In the mitochondria, it helps stabilize ATP molecules, supporting energy production. This stabilization is crucial because muscles require a constant supply of ATP to contract and relax properly - which is why it helps relieve muscle cramps, especially in women over 50. It also has a role to play in muscle relaxation and contraction by regulating calcium balance. Low magnesium levels can lead to excessive calcium in muscle cells, which causes prolonged contractions and cramps, usually due to the hormonal changes (lack of them) as we go through menopause.

Enzymes involved in glucose metabolism also need cofactors like chromium which helps the action of insulin on glucose (it helps the effective uptake of glucose by cells). Again, the decline in estrogen levels during and after menopause can affect the way the body processes glucose and insulin.

Antioxidant Production and Function

Selenium is a trace mineral and cofactor for the enzyme glutathione peroxidase. It is involved in several bodily functions, including antioxidant defense, thyroid function, and immune response. The enzyme helps detoxify harmful substances and protects cells from oxidative damage. After menopause, the decline in estrogen can lead to increased oxidative stress, as estrogen has antioxidant properties that help protect cells from damage.

This is an example of the cofactors which are essential for the proper function of enzymes involved in various processes in our cells, including energy production, glucose metabolism, and our antioxidant defense and, in particular, for women as estrogen levels fall.

Now, let's go back and look at cellular health and the main components that we are interested in.

The Role of Nutrients in Cellular Functions

Our body is composed of trillions of cells, each functioning as a mini-factory that carries out complex biochemical processes necessary for life.

These processes include producing energy, metabolizing glucose, and synthesizing antioxidants, which protect the body from oxidative stress and inflammation.

For these cellular factories to operate efficiently, they require a steady supply of nutrients. This is why maintaining a nutrient-rich diet, particularly one that supports cellular health and reduces inflammation is so important.

Energy Production

Mitochondria: Converts nutrients into adenosine triphosphate (ATP), the primary energy carrier in cells.
B vitamins, especially B1 (thiamine), B2 (riboflavin), B3 (niacin), B5 (pantothenic acid), and B6 (pyridoxine), play crucial roles in energy metabolism.
Magnesium acts as a cofactor in many ATP-generating reactions.

Glucose Metabolism

Insulin helps cells take in glucose from the blood to be used for energy.
Chromium enhances insulin's effectiveness, helping glucose metabolism.
Fiber-rich foods slow the absorption of sugar, helping to maintain stable blood glucose levels.

Antioxidant Production and Function

Vitamin C and **Vitamin E** are powerful antioxidants that protect cells from oxidative damage.
Selenium, the enzyme that helps detoxify harmful substances.

Polyphenols found in fruits, vegetables, and certain beverages like tea and red wine, exhibit strong antioxidant properties.

To make the most intermitting fasting you should aim to avoid inflammatory and insulin-resistance-promoting foods while including nutrient-rich, whole foods to support metabolic health.

While bad oils, refined sugars, and chemical additives can cause inflammation, disrupt hormone balance, and prevent the body's ability to efficiently metabolize food, whole foods rich in healthy fats and quality proteins, can support hormonal health, reduce inflammation, and deliver a more efficient and healthy metabolic state.

Reminder: Nutrient Balance and Why It Works

- Proteins: Essential for muscle repair and maintenance, especially important during intermittent fasting to help preserve lean mass and for those of us over 50.
- Carbohydrates: Focus on complex carbs like whole grains, fruits, and vegetables, which provide sustained energy and fiber for digestive health.
- Fats: Healthy fats from sources like avocados, nuts, and olive oil help in satiety, hormone production, and overall cellular health.
- Calories: The specific calorie intake can vary based on individual goals (weight maintenance, loss, or gain), but the emphasis is often on nutrient-dense foods within the eating window to support overall health and energy balance.

Key Vitamins and Why They're Important

Vitamin A: Important for vision, immune function, and skin health (found in vegetables like carrots and leafy greens).

Vitamin C: Essential for immune function, wound healing, and as an antioxidant (found in fruits like berries and citrus).

Vitamin D: Critical for bone health and immune function (found in eggs and fortified dairy products).

Vitamin E: Acts as an antioxidant, supports immune function, and skin health (found in nuts, seeds, and olive oil).

Vitamin K: Important for blood clotting and bone health (found in leafy greens like spinach and kale).

B Vitamins (B1, B2, B3, B6, B12): Essential for energy metabolism, nerve function, and red blood cell production (found in whole grains, lean meats, dairy, and leafy greens).

Fiber: Although not a vitamin, fiber is crucial for digestive health and can help manage blood sugar levels (found in whole grains, fruits, and vegetables)

Healthy Fats

These include olive oil, avocado oil, MCT oil, flaxseed oil, pumpkin seed oil, grass-fed butter, nut butters, olives, and avocados. Healthy fats are crucial for hormonal balance, snd overall health. They help stabilize blood sugar levels and can help the body to burn fat more efficiently.

Quality Proteins

Grass-fed beef, bison, turkey, chicken, pork, eggs, and certain charcuterie meats like salami and prosciutto are recommended. Quality proteins are essential for muscle maintenance, hormonal health, and satiety. They provide essential amino acids and can help manage hunger during fasting periods.

Nutrient-dense foods

Nutrient-dense food are all around us and they are those that provide a high amount of vitamins, minerals, and other beneficial substances with relatively few calories. They are essential for maintaining good health and can help prevent chronic diseases. Here are some examples of nutrient-dense foods:

Leafy Greens: Spinach, kale, swiss chard, and collard greens are rich in vitamins A, C, K, and folate, as well as fiber and antioxidants.

Berries: Blueberries, strawberries, raspberries, and blackberries are packed with vitamins, fiber, and antioxidants while being low in calories.

Nuts and Seeds: Almonds, chia seeds, flaxseeds, and walnuts provide healthy fats, protein, fiber, and essential minerals like magnesium and zinc.

Lean Proteins: Salmon, chicken breast, tofu, and legumes (beans, lentils, chickpeas) are excellent sources of protein, omega-3 fatty acids, and various vitamins and minerals.

Whole Grains: Quinoa, brown rice, oatmeal, and barley are high in fiber, B vitamins, and essential minerals like iron and magnesium.

Cruciferous Vegetables: Broccoli, Brussels sprouts, cauliflower, and cabbage offer fiber, vitamins C and K, and several antioxidants.

Colorful Vegetables: Bell peppers, carrots, tomatoes, and sweet potatoes are rich in vitamins, fiber, and phytonutrients.
Fruits: Oranges, apples, bananas, and kiwi provide a variety of vitamins, fiber, and antioxidants.

Dairy or Alternatives: Greek yogurt, kefir, and fortified plant-based milks (almond, soy, oat) are good sources of calcium, protein, and probiotics.

Herbs and Spices: Turmeric, ginger, garlic, and cinnamon are not only flavorful but also provide antioxidants and anti-inflammatory compounds.

Antioxidants

If, like me, you are particularly interested in which foods are antioxidants, here are some examples.

Fruits

- Berries (blueberries, strawberries, raspberries, blackberries)
- Citrus fruits (oranges, lemons, grapefruits)
- Apples, plums, and grapes

Vegetables

- Leafy greens (spinach, kale)
- Broccoli and Brussels sprouts
- Carrots and sweet potatoes

Nuts and Seeds

- Almonds, walnuts, and pecans
- Sunflower seeds and chia seeds

Beverages

- Green tea and black tea
- Coffee
- Red wine (in moderation)

Others

- Dark chocolate, Whole grains, Legumes (beans, lentils)

A day's diet under intermittent fasting can vary based on personal preferences and dietary goals, but here's an example of a balanced approach that includes a good mix of nutrients, fats, carbs, calories, and proteins.

Plan a Day's Meal Incorporating Nutrient-Dense Foods

Breakfast

Green Smoothie Bowl: Blend spinach, kale, a banana, a handful of blueberries, and almond milk. Top with chia seeds, flaxseeds, and a few slices of kiwi.

Mid-Morning Snack

Greek Yogurt with Berries: A cup of Greek yogurt topped with a mix of strawberries, raspberries, and a drizzle of honey.

Lunch

Quinoa Salad: A quinoa base with chopped bell peppers, cherry tomatoes, cucumbers, chickpeas, and a handful of spinach. Dress with olive oil, lemon juice, and a sprinkle of sunflower seeds.

Afternoon Snack

Apple Slices with Almond Butter: Sliced apple served with a tablespoon of almond butter.

Dinner

Grilled Salmon with Sweet Potato and Broccoli: A portion of grilled salmon served with roasted sweet potato wedges and steamed broccoli. Add a side salad with mixed greens, carrots, and a light vinaigrette.

Tea

Turmeric Ginger Tea: A soothing tea made with fresh turmeric, ginger, and a touch of honey.

This meal plan incorporates a variety of nutrient-dense foods that provide a balanced intake of vitamins, minerals, fiber, healthy fats, and protein and focuses on whole foods that support overall health and well-being.

There are lots of online resources and recipe books that can help you work out the make-up of your food - the calories, carbs, protein amount and so on - that will help you build your ideal menu.

Getting started

It's a great idea to prepare for your fasting by spending no less than a week (the ideal timeframe is 2 weeks, but choose whatever works for you) adjusting your diet, getting familiar with what's in what you eat, and replacing unhealthy with healthy foods. Try to start by filling it out at least 7 days of a food diary - included next, to get you into the habit of thinking about what is in the food that you are eating.

It's now time to take stock and think about your diet - we'll discuss lifestyle next.

We have talked about the balance of calories, protein, carbs, fats and nutrients. Every change begins by being aware of what you eat. The very best way to do this, is to begin tracking what you do and what you put into your body.

In the following pages we have a weeks-worth of nutrient trackers. Fill them in, it will really help you to begin to know what you are eating and being conscious of it but before then, here is an idea of what you want to consider and an example of some daily meals.

Exercise

- Check the labels to see what's in your food and remember that shifting towards whole, nutrient-dense foods can significantly help combat obesity.

- Assess the nutritional quality and suitability of your current diet.

- Gradually eliminate processed foods and replace them with whole, nutrient-dense alternatives.

- Incorporate stress management techniques such as mindfulness, exercise, or hobbies into your daily routine.

Before you begin: Exercises and Reflective Questions

Rethinking the Role of Calories

Question: Think about the last time you were on a diet. Did you get stressed? How has your perception of calories influenced your dieting choices? What new understanding do you have about calories now?

_____

_____

_____

_____

Action: Research and list foods that are nutrient-dense rather than just low in calories. Plan a day's meal incorporating these foods.

_____

_____

_____

_____

Identifying Toxic Ingredients

Question: Are you aware of 'obesogens' or other harmful ingredients in your food and environment? How might they be affecting your health?

Action: Go through your pantry and read the labels of your food items. Research any unknown ingredients to determine if they could be harmful. Make a plan to replace items with healthier alternatives.

My Exposure to Toxins

Analyzing Past Dieting Experiences

Question: Think about your past dieting attempts. In what ways might they have conflicted with your body's natural processes?

Action: Write down a list of diets you have tried in the past. Next to each, note any negative effects you experienced. Reflect on how these diets might have been at odds with your body's needs.

Diet Name: _____

Negative Impacts

_____

_____

_____

Diet Name: _____

Negative Impacts

_____

_____

_____

Practical Diet Guide to Intermittent Fasting For Women Over 50

Diet Name: _____

Negative Impacts

Diet Name: _____

Negative Impacts

Other Notes:

Foods to Eat

What is your body trying to tell you?

Question: Think about the last time you felt unwell or fatigued. What could your body have been trying to say to you?

Understanding Cellular Health and Nutrition

Question: Reflect on your current diet. Are there specific nutrients you think you might be lacking based on what you've learned about cellular health? You can come back to this later.

Action: Start a food diary to understand your calorie and nutrient intake and identify gaps. An example dairy to track your Calorie Quality and Nutrition intake is included on the following page. Use this as a guide to prompt you to think about what you eat and to help you get into the habit of finding the information that you really want to track, such as calories, carbs, fat content, proteins and vitamins and minerals. There are five bank diary nutrition pages that you can use to get into the hang of it. It follows as the end of this section.

After reading the book and completing this workbook, compare this with a list of essential nutrients for cellular health.

Here is another, more specific, example of daily meal plan that might help to get you started. Add in the nutrient amounts of each highlighted on the following pages by following the example.

Chapter 8

Example Menu

Example Daily Diet

Morning (During Fasting Period)

Water, Herbal Tea, or Black Coffee: These are typically allowed during the fasting period as they are low in calories and can help curb hunger.

Hydrating and low in calories. Coffee provides some antioxidants.

Break-Fast (First Meal of the Day)

Time: Around mid-morning to early afternoon, depending on your fasting window.

Meal Options:

- Protein Source: Eggs (scrambled or boiled), Greek yogurt, or

a protein smoothie (with protein powder). For vitamin D (eggs).
- Carbohydrates: Whole-grain toast or oats (steel-cut or rolled) with berries or a banana. Whole-grain toast or oats for fiber and B vitamins.
- Healthy Fats: Avocado slices on toast, or nuts (such as almonds or walnuts) added to yogurt or smoothie. Avocado slices for vitamin E and monounsaturated fats.

Lunch

Time: Around midday to early afternoon.

Meal Options:

- Protein Source: Grilled chicken breast, tofu, or fish (like salmon). Grilled chicken breast for B vitamins.
- Vegetables: Large salad with mixed greens, tomatoes, cucumbers, and bell peppers for vitamins A, C, and K.
- Complex Carbohydrates: Quinoa or brown rice for fiber and B vitamins.
- Healthy Fats: Olive oil-based dressing on the salad, or avocado slices for vitamin E.

Afternoon Snack

Time: Mid-afternoon.

Snack Options:

- Protein: Cottage cheese (protein and calcium) or a small handful of nuts (like almonds or walnuts).
- Fruits: Apple slices or a small serving of berries for vitamin C and antioxidants.

Example Menu

Dinner

Time: Early evening, typically before the end of the feeding window.

Meal Options:

- Protein Source: Lean meat (such as lean beef or turkey), or legumes (like lentils or chickpeas for a vegetarian option) for B vitamins.
- Vegetables: Steamed broccoli, carrots, and bell peppers. Steamed broccoli and carrots for vitamins A, C, and K.
- Complex Carbohydrates: Sweet potatoes or whole-grain pasta. Sweet potatoes for fiber, vitamin A, and potassium.
- Healthy Fats: A drizzle of olive oil on vegetables or a small serving of avocado for vitamin E.

Evening Snack (Optional)

Time: Closer to the end of the feeding window, if desired.

Snack Options:

- Protein: A small serving of cottage cheese (probiotics) or a protein-rich snack like a hard-boiled egg
- Fats and Carbohydrates: A handful of nuts (like almonds or walnuts for vitamin E and healthy fats) with a piece of fruit.

Nutrient Diary - example only

Meal	Food Item	Cals - kcal	Carbs (g)	Protein (g)	Fats (g)	Vitamins/Minerals
Breakfast	2 eggs, wholegrain toast, orange juice	350	35g (toast juice)	14g - mostly eggs	14g - mostly from eggs	A, D, E, B12 (from eggs); C (from juice)
Morning Snack	Greek Yogurt (150g), Almonds (28g)	250	15g	15g	15g	Calcium (from yogurt), E, Magnesium (from almonds)
Lunch	Grilled Chicken (100g), greens, cherry tomatoes, cucumbers, olive oil and vinegar dressing)	350	10	25g	20g - mostly from dressing	A, C, K (from greens), Antioxidants
Afternoon Snack	Apple, Dark Choco-late (1 ounce)	150	30g (most from apple)	2g	8g (from chocolate)	C (from apple), Iron (from chocolate)
Dinner	150 g Grilled Salmon, 1/2 Cup Cooked Quinoa, Steamed Broccoli (1 cup)	500	20g	40g	25g (mostly from salmon)	Omega-3 (from salmon), B Vitamins, Iron, K (from quinoa and broccoli)
Herbal Tea	0	0	0	0	0	0

Nutrient Diary: Date: Day:

Meal	Food Item	Cals-kcal	Carbs (g)	Protein (g)	Fats (g)	Vitamins/Minerals

Nutrient Diary: Date: Day:

Meal	Food Item	Cals-kcal	Carbs (g)	Protein (g)	Fats (g)	Vitamins/Minerals

Nutrient Diary: Date: Day:

Meal	Food Item	Cals-kcal	Carbs (g)	Protein (g)	Fats (g)	Vitamins/Minerals

Nutrient Diary: Date: Day:

Meal	Food Item	Cals-kcal	Carbs (g)	Protein (g)	Fats (g)	Vitamins/Minerals

Nutrient Diary: Date: Day:

Meal	Food Item	Cals-kcal	Carbs (g)	Protein (g)	Fats (g)	Vitamins/Minerals

Nutrient Diary: Date: Day:

Meal	Food Item	Cals-kcal	Carbs (g)	Protein (g)	Fats (g)	Vitamins/Minerals

Nutrient Diary: Date: Day:

Meal	Food Item	Cals-kcal	Carbs (g)	Protein (g)	Fats (g)	Vitamins/Minerals

Chapter 9

Goals and Fasting Types

We have mentioned the vagus nerve earlier, and it includes work to reduce stress and anxiety including practices such as meditating, which can help us understand our brings 'why'. It can help you focus on what it is you are trying to achieve and why you are aiming for that goal. Be honest with yourself and most of all believe that you can do this. You can.

For example, your reason might be weight loss, hormonal balance, or to address a specific health condition. Or it might be simply for general health and to improve your metabolic rate to take a preventative approach.

The fasting method you choose and the food that you eat can all have a different focus in order to target your desired outcome.

In my case, I am over 50, post menopausal and wanted to generally improve my health and target inflammation (with oxidative stress a part of that) with the goal of establishing a healthy diet now, so that I can be fit and healthy into my old age - and enjoy my retirement to the full! This is just an example, but try to have a big goal so that you know what it might mean for you.

There are lots of reason to consider intermittent fasting, and some of these are detailed below along with the type of diet plan that can work for each objective. Just remember to vary your diet to improve gut health and reduce cravings.

If you have health conditions like PCOS or are in menopause, pay close attention to how your body responds to dietary changes in carbohydrates and fats.

Improving Gut Health

Goal: Improve gut health to reduce inflammation

Fasting helps reset the gut microbiome, promoting the growth of beneficial bacteria which helps manage inflammation.

Recommended Foods (especially when ending your fast) : Fermented foods (like yogurt, kefir, sauerkraut, kimchi), prebiotic-rich foods (like garlic, onions, leeks, asparagus), and fiber-rich foods (like fruits, vegetables, and whole grains).

Building Muscle

Goal: Support muscle growth and repair after fasting.

For those looking to build muscle, breaking a fast with high-protein foods can support muscle repair and growth - we'll cover how to break a fast in more detail in a later chapter. This isn't just a great fast for athletes but is for anyone engaged in strength training.

High-protein foods (like lean meats, fish, eggs, dairy products, legumes, and protein shakes), and foods with healthy fats (like avocados, nuts, and seeds) to provide sustained energy and support overall nutrition.

Burning Fat

Goal: Promote fat loss and improve metabolic health.

Recommended Foods: Low-carbohydrate foods (like leafy greens, non-starchy vegetables, and healthy fats), lean proteins (like chicken, turkey, and fish), and foods that are high in healthy fats (like avocados, nuts, seeds, and olive oil). Avoiding sugary and high-carb foods can help maintain a state of ketosis, where the body burns fat for fuel.

General Health and Tasty Food

Goal: Enjoy a variety of foods that satisfy personal cravings and preferences while still being mindful of health.

Recommended Foods: A balanced mix of foods that include a variety of fruits, vegetables, proteins, and whole grains. This approach emphasizes enjoyment and moderation, allowing for a wider range of foods while still focusing on overall health.

What is your goal?

We'll do this again, but have a go now at writing down what sprints to mind. Don't overthink it!

Type of Fast

Various intermittent fasting methods differ in their fasting and eating windows, offering benefits suited for different health goals. I am going to summarise the most common ones below, but will go on to only focus on two to get you started. It's useful to know what they are, so that you can move onto these if you decide you want to and once you get used to buying and cooking the food that your body needs - and, of course, already seeing the results.

1. Spontaneous Meal Skipping

Structure: Skip meals when convenient without following a strict schedule.
Example: Skip breakfast if not hungry, eat lunch and dinner as usual.

Benefits:

- Flexible and easy to adapt.
- Reduces calorie intake naturally.
- Encourages intuitive eating habits.

Good For: Individuals with unpredictable schedules or those who prefer a less rigid approach but lack of structure may make it hard to stick to or benefit from.

When Not to Do It:

- People who need regular meals to maintain blood sugar levels.
- Those prone to overeating later in the day.

2. 12/12 Method

Structure: Fast for 12 hours and eat within a 12-hour window.
Example: Eat between 8 AM and 8 PM, fast from 8 PM to 8 AM.

Benefits:

- Gentle introduction to fasting.
- Steady improvement in metabolic markers.
- Easier on the digestive system.

Good For: Beginners and those looking to establish a healthier eating schedule. Very easy to start and maintain.

When Not to Do It:

Generally safe for most people, but individuals with specific medical conditions should consult a doctor.

3. 16/8 Method

Structure: Fast for 16 hours and eat within an 8-hour window.
Example: Eat between 12 PM and 8 PM, fast from 8 PM to 12 PM the next day.
Benefits:

- Supports weight loss and fat loss: Effective due to reduced eating window.
- Weight Loss and insulin sensitivity: Improved by regular fasting periods.
- Ease of Use: Fits well into daily life, minimal disruption.

Good For: Beginners, those seeking gradual weight loss, and people with busy schedules.

When Not to Do It:

- People with hypoglycemia or diabetes who need regular meals.
- Individuals with a history of eating disorders.
- Those who experience extreme hunger or fatigue during fasting periods.

4. 5/2 Method

Structure: Eat normally for five days a week and restrict calorie intake to 500-600 calories on two non-consecutive days.
Example: Normal eating Monday-Friday, 500-600 calories on Tuesday and Thursday.
Benefits:

- Significant calorie reduction on fasting days.
- Fasting days may boost cognitive function.
- Normal eating most days, easier social engagements.
- Easy to maintain social eating habits on non-fasting days.

Good For: Those who prefer not to fast daily but still want health benefits.

When Not to Do It:

- Individuals with a history of eating disorders.
- Those who find calorie restriction days excessively stressful or difficult.
- People with certain medical conditions needing consistent nutrient intake.

5. Eat-Stop-Eat

Structure: Fast for 24 hours once or twice a week.
Example: Eat dinner at 7 PM, fast until 7 PM the next day.
Benefits:

- Significant caloric reduction.
- Longer fasting may enhance metabolism and boost metabolic rate
- Boosts metabolic rate.
- Longer fasts promoting cellular repair (autophagy)

Good For: Individuals comfortable with longer fasting periods and those seeking substantial weight loss. It requires mental discipline for 24-hour fasts.

When Not to Do It:

- Individuals who have never fasted before.
- People with blood sugar regulation issues.
- Those who may experience severe hunger or fatigue.

6. Alternate-Day Fasting

Structure: Alternate between days of normal eating and fasting.
Example: Eat normally on Monday, fast or consume 500-600 calories on Tuesday, repeat.

Benefits:

- Effective for weight loss and fat loss.
- May improve heart health and reduce inflammation.

Good For: Individuals who can handle regular fasting days and want quick results but demands regular adherence.

When Not to Do It:

- Individuals with demanding physical jobs or high-energy needs.
- People prone to binge eating on non-fasting days.
- Those with certain medical conditions requiring regular nutrient intake.

7. Warrior Diet

Structure: Eat small amounts of raw fruits and vegetables during the day and one large meal at night within a 4-hour window.

Example: Eat a large meal between 6 PM and 10 PM.

Benefits:

- Mimics ancestral eating patterns (delivering hormonal balance)
- May enhance nutrient absorption.
- Large evening meal may improve muscle recovery.

Good For: Those who prefer to eat one large meal later at night and can handle extended fasting periods. It has a strict eating window.

When Not to Do It:

- Individuals needing regular meals for energy (e.g., athletes).
- People who may overeat or binge during the eating window.
- Those with digestive issues exacerbated by large meals.

While all of the methods can help with weight loss, improve metabolic health, and reduce inflammation, choosing the right approach depends on your own individual needs and how well it fits into your daily routine.

For women over 50 longer fasts don't tend to be recommended so if you are thinking about a longer fasting window (beyond 16:8, but certainly beyond 5:2) then check with your health care provider.

As we have seen, combining intermittent fasting with a nutrient-rich, anti-inflammatory diet can amplify the results so make sure to include as much as you can. Don't forget that reducing inflammation can help conditions like arthritis and asthma (partly due to reduced oxidative stress and improved insulin sensitivity - which intermittent fasting helps with).

It goes without saying that intermittent fasting will no be suitable for everyone. For example if you are pregnant or breastfeeding then your nutrient demands are higher, as is the case for children and adolescents who are growing and developing.

It can trigger disordered eating patterns in those with a history of eating disorders, while anyone already underweight should avoid any further weight loss.

And those with medical conditions like diabetes, low blood pressure, or other health issues should consult a healthcare provider before starting intermittent fasting as should anyone experiencing extreme stress or fatigue.

Chapter 10

Women, Hormones and Glucose

Having looked at the basic food and nutrients that we need - and why, now would be a good time to consider different strategies at different times of the month - and specifically our hormones. While hormones don't impact men in the same way as women, we will touch on this too.

Women cycle every 28 days and the central point at which everything centers is ovulation - which happens in the middle of the 28-day cycle. During the first 14 days, you make more estrogen (estradiol) than progesterone; after ovulation, you make more progesterone than estrogen. An ovulatory cycle is when you make both progesterone and estrogen, and ovulation occurs.

An anovulatory cycle means no ovulation occurs, and therefore, no progesterone has been produced - this is because progesterone is only made as a result of ovulation. It is also the anovulatory cycle that is most common during peri-menopause, as progesterone production slowly falls through each missed cycle.

Estrogen, progesterone (and, to a lesser degree, testosterone) fluctuate wildly during peri-menopause. It is the imbalance and falls in levels of these hormones that affect our mood, anxiety, sleep, bones, mental health, weight, and so on - more-or-less all of the experiences you will have to some degree or another before, during, and after menopause.

The hormone fluctuations reduce the body's ability to control the metabolic rate, causing an increased risk of obesity, high blood pressure, insulin resistance, high cholesterol levels, type 2 diabetes, and Alzheimer's disease.

Weight gain during menopause is due to the declining levels of estrogen and, in post-menopausal women this combined with decreasing physical activity levels and an increase in the intake of unhealthy foods often the result of 'growing up' life events such as becoming an empty nester.

Why Intermittent Fasting is Often Considered for Women

Given these hormonal changes and their effects on metabolism, intermittent fasting is often considered a beneficial strategy for women, especially during peri-menopause and menopause.

It can help improve insulin sensitivity, which is often compromised during hormonal fluctuations. Better insulin sensitivity helps regulate blood sugar levels and can prevent weight gain associated with insulin resistance. As we know it also helps metabolic switching, where the body shifts from using glucose to burning stored fats for energy. This is particularly useful for women experiencing weight gain due to hormonal changes.

Reduced levels of insulin can help balance other hormones such as estrogen and progesterone which can reduce symptoms like mood swings, anxiety, and sleep disturbances.

Because fasting can lower inflammation levels in the body, and since chronic inflammation is linked to many of the health issues made worse by hormonal imbalances, intermittent fasting can be a powerful tool in managing these conditions.

Many women also report improved mental clarity and stabilized mood when fasting, likely due to the combined effects of improved metabolic health and hormonal balance.

The First 14 Days of the Cycle

During the first 14 days of your cycle, when estrogen levels are higher, you might find that you have more energy and a higher tolerance for physical activity. This phase, known as the follicular phase, is an excellent time to incorporate higher intensity workouts and strength training. Your body is more insulin-sensitive during this phase, so it's also a good time to consume complex carbohydrates and lean proteins, which can support muscle growth and recovery from exercise. Intermittent fasting during this phase can be more comfortable and effective due to higher energy levels and better metabolic flexibility.

Adjustments for Last 14 Days of the Cycle

In the last 14 days of your cycle, after ovulation, progesterone levels increase, and you enter the luteal phase. During this phase, you might experience lower energy levels and increased cravings. It's essential to listen to your body and adjust your fasting and exercise routines accordingly. Lower-intensity exercises like yoga, walking, and swimming can be more appropriate during this time. Nutritionally, focus on healthy fats and proteins to stabilize blood sugar levels and help manage cravings. You may also consider shortening your fasting window or incorporating more nutrient-dense foods to ensure your body gets the support it needs during this phase.

Action Plans

Start Tracking: Begin by tracking your menstrual cycle to identify the 2 broad parts of your cycle (first 14 and last 14 days).

Plan Your Fasting: Schedule longer fasts during the first part of your cycle and shorter fasts or dietary considerations during the second half. You can break down your phases in more detail later but this is a great way to start. Follow the 12:12 plan and the actions that follow for women over 50.

Menopause and Beyond

If you are over 50 you may already either find yourself at menopause or 'post menopause'. So what does this mean for intermittent fasting and how can it specifically help?

Menopause is the natural biological process marking the end of menstrual cycles, typically diagnosed after you've gone 12 months without a menstrual period. The transition to menopause, known as peri-menopause, involves significant hormonal changes, particularly the decline in estrogen and progesterone levels.

Post-Menopause (the period of life after you have experienced 12 consecutive months without a menstrual period) is a time when your body is continuing to adapt to these lower hormone levels, and it can - and does - affect various aspects of health, including metabolism, bone density, and cardiovascular health.

Intermittent Fasting for Women Over 50

Intermittent fasting can offer several health benefits for women over 50, particularly in managing the changes and challenges associated with menopause and post-menopause:

1. Weight Management: Hormonal changes during menopause can lead to weight gain, especially around the abdomen. As we already know, intermittent fasting helps weight loss by increasing fat burning and improving metabolic health.

2. Improved Insulin Sensitivity: The decline in estrogen levels during menopause can lead to insulin resistance, and along with the impact on glucose absorption, it can increase the risk of type 2 diabetes. Intermittent fasting has been shown to improve insulin sensitivity, helping to stabilize blood sugar levels and reduce the risk of diabetes.

3. Enhanced Metabolism: As we age, our metabolic rate naturally slows down. As well as the other metabolic effects, intermittent fasting can boost the production of norepinephrine, a hormone that increases fat burning. Additionally, it can help maintain muscle mass, which is crucial for a healthy metabolism.

4. Reduced Inflammation: Chronic inflammation is a concern for many postmenopausal women and is linked to various age-related diseases. Because intermittent fasting can reduce markers of inflammation in the body, it can lower risk of inflammatory diseases.

5. Heart Health: Post-menopausal women are at a higher risk of cardiovascular diseases due to changes in lipid profiles and increased oxidative stress. Intermittent fasting can improve heart health by lowering blood pressure, reducing cholesterol levels, and decreasing oxidative stress.

6. Improved Cognitive Function: The risk of cognitive decline increases with age and hormonal changes during menopause can impact brain health. Because intermittent fasting promotes the production of brain-derived neurotrophic factor (BDNF), which we met earlier, it may also protect against neurodegenerative diseases like Alzheimer's (due to its support of neuron growth and subsequent cognitive function).

7. Bone Health: Bone density can decrease significantly after menopause due to lower estrogen levels, increasing the risk of osteoporosis. While intermittent fasting alone is not a treatment for bone health, combined with a nutrient-dense diet rich in calcium and vitamin D, it can support overall bone health and reduce the risk of fractures.

It was quite a surprise for me to discover that many of the benefits of intermittent fasting were ideal for women over 50 - and specifically around the effects of reduced estrogen. The key highlights for me were that it helps to manage weight, improve insulin sensitivity, and reduce inflammation. All of which can lead to a healthier, longer, and happier life.

Action Plans

Start Gradually: Begin with a 12:12 fasting schedule (12 hours of fasting and 12 hours of eating) to allow your body to adapt. After a week or two, gradually increase to a 16:8 schedule (16 hours of fasting and 8 hours of eating).

Track Your Progress: Use a journal, an app or that logs provided later in the book to track your fasting hours, eating windows, and how you feel throughout the process. Note any changes in energy levels, mood, and physical health.

Plan Balanced Meals: During your eating windows, focus on nutrient-dense meals. Include lean proteins, healthy fats, whole grains, and plenty of fruits and vegetables to ensure you get essential vitamins and minerals.

Stay Hydrated: Drink plenty of water throughout the day, especially during fasting periods. You can also include herbal teas or black coffee if you prefer.

Listen to Your Body: Pay attention to how your body responds to fasting. If you feel overly fatigued or unwell, adjust your fasting schedule or consult with a healthcare provider.

Include Physical Activity: Incorporate regular physical activity into your routine. This can include walking, yoga, strength training, or any other form of exercise you enjoy. Remember, exercise can help improve insulin sensitivity and overall health.

Focus on Sleep: Ensure you get adequate sleep each night. It is essential for overall health and can help your body adapt to intermittent fasting.

Monitor Health Metrics: Regularly check important health metrics such as blood sugar levels, blood pressure, and weight. This will help you track the impact of intermittent fasting on your health.

Complete the month planner as a guide to help you think about how to plan your fasts. If your objective is weight loss, don't forget to add your weight and waist measurements at the start and end of each month.

Chapter 11

Men, Hormones and Andropause

It's not only women who can experience the effects of hormone loss as they age, men too can also experience a variety of health changes, some of which are hormone-related. Here are just some common symptoms and conditions that can affect men's health as they age.

Common Symptoms and Conditions

1. Decreased Testosterone Levels (Andropause)

- Symptoms: Fatigue, depression, reduced libido, erectile dysfunction, decreased muscle mass, increased body fat, and reduced bone density.
- Hormone-Related: Yes. Testosterone levels typically decline about 1% per year after age 30.

2. Prostate Health Issues

- Symptoms: Frequent urination, difficulty starting and stopping urination, weak urine stream, and nocturia (frequent urination at night).
- Hormone-Related: Indirectly. Prostate enlargement (Benign Prostatic Hyperplasia, BPH) is influenced by hormones like dihydrotestosterone (DHT).

3. Cardiovascular Disease

- Symptoms: Chest pain, shortness of breath, dizziness, fatigue, and irregular heartbeats.
- Hormone-Related: Can be influenced by hormone levels, including testosterone, which affects cholesterol metabolism and vascular health.

4. Osteoporosis and Bone Density Loss

- Symptoms: Increased risk of fractures, back pain, and loss of height.
- Hormone-Related: Yes. Testosterone plays a role in maintaining bone density.

5. Metabolic Changes

- Symptoms: Weight gain, especially around the abdomen, insulin resistance, and type 2 diabetes.
- Hormone-Related: Partially. Hormones like testosterone and growth hormone influence body composition and metabolism.

6. Mood Changes and Depression

- Symptoms: Persistent sadness, loss of interest in activities, changes in sleep patterns, and irritability.
- Hormone-Related: Yes. Lower testosterone levels can contribute to mood changes and depression.

7. Sexual Dysfunction

- Symptoms: Erectile dysfunction, reduced libido, and fertility issues.
- Hormone-Related: Yes. Declining testosterone levels are directly linked to these symptoms.

Andropause, sometimes referred to as male menopause, is characterized by the gradual decline in testosterone levels in men, typically starting in their late 40s to early 50s.

Unlike female menopause, where hormone production drops rapidly, andropause occurs more gradually and with more varied symptoms. Here are some key points about andropause:

- **Hormonal Decline**: The primary hormone involved is testosterone, but other hormones like DHEA and growth hormone also decline with age.
- **Symptoms**: Include many of the common conditions listed above, such as decreased libido, erectile dysfunction, fatigue, depression, and loss of muscle mass.
- **Management**: Lifestyle changes (diet, exercise), hormone replacement therapy (HRT), and medications can help manage symptoms.

Parallels to Menopause

While there are similarities between andropause and menopause, there are also key differences:

- **Onset**: Menopause typically occurs abruptly in women around age 50, while andropause is a gradual decline over many years.
- **Symptoms**: Both can involve mood changes, sexual dysfunction, and changes in physical health, but the specific symptoms and their severity can differ.
- **Hormone Therapy**: HRT is commonly used to manage symptoms of menopause, and testosterone replacement therapy (TRT) can be used for andropause, although TRT is more controversial due to its potential risks.

Chapter 12

Fasting Planning

Our objective is to be healthy, and in many, but not all, cases to loose weight. The wonderful thing about intermittent fasting is that it can not only help use lose weight - and keep it off - but the wider health benefits are in themselves worth it.

To summarise the last few pages, it can improve our gut health and mitochondria - the gut-brain connection - improving our brain and mental health, reducing stress, not only in our cells and body but the stress that effects our mental health which leads to sleepless nights and anxiety, as well as - along with many of organs including our liver.

It can change our metabolic set-point, making it easier for us to stick to the balanced food intake that or body needs.

The anti-inflammatory benefits are one of my favourites.

It can help our cells get rid of the things they don't want or needs and that damage them, keeping them healthy and better able to regenerate other healthy cells (rather than unhealthy cells - these are the ones that often cause cancer).

However, before you jump right in, you need to begin slowly. Find out what works for you. Don't over-do it and work on all of your health - including your mind. Read, explore and research and begin understanding what you are giving your body right now.

So now I will give you two great examples. The first is perfect to start with - its the 12:12 diet and then I will give you an example of how to approach the 16:8.

Starting with a 12:12 fasting plan and gradually building up to a 16:8 fasting plan is a practical and sustainable approach supported by scientific evidence. It involves fasting for 12 hours and having a 12-hour eating window. This approach is generally easier for beginners as it aligns closely with natural eating patterns and the body's circadian rhythms.

It allows your body to adapt gradually, reducing the risk of hunger and energy issues, and increasing the likelihood of long-term success. Even a 12-hour fasting period can help regulate blood sugar, help with weight management levels and improve insulin sensitivity while matching eating patterns with the body's natural circadian rhythm can help to improve sleep and overall metabolic health. It can also help establish a routine that can be gradually extended to 12, 14, 15 add finally 16 hours.

Once again, try and note down what you eat now, think about the food you want to eat and like (and what it does for you), then plan what you want to buy as you get ready to start. Start removing inflammatory foods and incorporating healthier options.

Ending a Fast

Ending a fast isn't just about eating or not eating but involves a planned approach based on your own health goals and build this in to your plan as you get used to it and learn more about how you react (and your goals).

There are a number of ways you can break a fast, each catering to different health objectives. For example resetting the microbiome, building muscle, or burning fat.

Reset Your Microbiome: Start incorporating probiotic, prebiotic, and polyphenol-rich foods into your first meal post-fasting.

Build Muscle: Post-fasting, focus on protein-rich foods, especially after strength training.

Burn Fat: Include healthy fats in your diet post-fasting to continue fat burning.

There is month planner after the 16/8 guide and before the 5/2 example.

Action Plans

Blood Sugar Monitoring: Regularly check your blood sugar levels after breaking your fast to understand its impact.

Personal Experimentation: Try different fasted snacks, foods and drinks and observe their effects on your fasting period.

Metabolic Flexibility and Adaptation: Note any changes that you notice to your body's ability to efficiently switch between different energy sources over time.

Dietary Guidelines: Try to remove harmful oils, refined sugars, flours, and chemicals from your diet.

Biometric Monitoring: Ideally, and over time. start using tools like glucose and ketone monitors to track bodily responses to fasting.

Education and Awareness: Continue learning about fasting, gut health, and insulin resistance to make even better decisions about your diet and fasting routine.

Goal Setting

Short-term Goals

- Successfully complete the one or two-week preparation phase.
- Eliminate specific harmful foods from your diet within the next week.

Long-term Goals

- Complete the 30-Day 12/12 plan and get to know what fasting window can work for a further stage (11,10,9 or 8)
- Develop a sustainable fasting routine as part of my lifestyle.

Action Plans example

For the Preparation Phase:

- Remove all harmful oils and refined foods from my kitchen.
- Plan meals that incorporate healthy fats and proteins.
- Gradually adjust meal times to compress the eating window.

During the 30-Day Plan

- Follow the daily fasting schedule strictly.
- Monitor and track weekly progress and how you feel.

Post-30 Day Plan

- Evaluate the impact on health and well-being.
- Integrate the most beneficial aspects of the reset into my regular diet.

Fasting Planning

Write your action plan here and note what you need to do to make them happen.

For the Preparation Phase (see the next few pages for a 14 day plan)

During the 30-Day Diet Plan for 12/12

Post-30 Days

Practical Diet Guide to Intermittent Fasting For Women Over 50

Fasting Planning

Preparation Phase: Paying attention to your menstrual cycle (for women) note what you intend to do over 4 weeks.

Day 1 Day/Date:

Menstrual Phase:
Eating Style/Goal:
Fast time start:
Fast time end:
Fast duration:

Food/meals/ingredients required from grocery store:

_____

_____

_____

_____

Practical Diet Guide to Intermittent Fasting For Women Over 50

Day 2 Day/Date:

Menstrual Phase:
Eating Style/Goal:
Fast time start:
Fast time end:
Fast duration:

Food/meals/ingredients required from grocery store

Fasting Planning

Day 3 Day/Date:

Menstrual Phase:
Eating Style/Goal:
Fast time start:
Fast time end:
Fast duration:

Food/meals/ingredients required from grocery store:

Practical Diet Guide to Intermittent Fasting For Women Over 50

Day 4 Day/Date:

Menstrual Phase:
Eating Style/Goal:
Fast time start:
Fast time end:
Fast duration:

Food/meals/ingredients required from grocery store

Day 5 Day/Date:

Menstrual Phase:
Eating Style/Goal:
Fast time start:
Fast time end:
Fast duration:

Food/meals/ingredients required from grocery store:

Day 6 Day/Date:

Menstrual Phase:
Eating Style/Goal:
Fast time start:
Fast time end:
Fast duration:

Food/meals/ingredients required from grocery store

Fasting Planning

Day 7 Day/Date:

Menstrual Phase:
Eating Style/Goal:
Fast time start:
Fast time end:
Fast duration:

Food/meals/ingredients required from grocery store:

Day 8 Day/Date:

Menstrual Phase:
Eating Style/Goal:
Fast time start:
Fast time end:
Fast duration:

Food/meals/ingredients required from grocery store

Fasting Planning

Day 9 Day/Date:

Menstrual Phase:
Eating Style/Goal:
Fast time start:
Fast time end:
Fast duration:

Food/meals/ingredients required from grocery store

Day 10 Day/Date:

Menstrual Phase:
Eating Style/Goal:
Fast time start:
Fast time end:
Fast duration:

Food/meals/ingredients required from grocery store

Day 11 Day/Date:

Menstrual Phase:
Eating Style/Goal:
Fast time start:
Fast time end:
Fast duration:

Food/meals/ingredients required from grocery store

Day 12 Day/Date:

Menstrual Phase:
Eating Style/Goal:
Fast time start:
Fast time end:
Fast duration:

Food/meals/ingredients required from grocery store

Fasting Planning

Day 13 Day/Date:

Menstrual Phase:
Eating Style/Goal:
Fast time start:
Fast time end:
Fast duration:

Food/meals/ingredients required from grocery store

Day 14 Day/Date:

Menstrual Phase:
Eating Style/Goal:
Fast time start:
Fast time end:
Fast duration:

Food/meals/ingredients required from grocery store

During the 30-day plan:

- Begin to vary your food and drink and take note of you you feel.
- Measure you BMR if you can.

Notes:

Chapter 13

The 12:12 Kick-start 30-Day Plan

This 30-day meal plan incorporates low and medium glycemic index (GI) foods, nutrient-dense ingredients, and essential vitamins and minerals to support overall health and manage blood sugar levels. The plan includes periods for breaking the fast and considerations for sustaining the diet. This is only an example to aim for if you wish to. You can stay at 12:12 or slowly increase your fasting window, but only do what you feel comfortable with.

I have left some space for you to take notes of meals you have prepared or thoughts or comments to add for yourself to review at a later date.

The 12:12 Kick-start 30-Day Plan

Daily Structure

Fasting Window: 8:00 PM - 8:00 AM (12 hours)

Eating Window: 8:00 AM - 8:00 PM (12 hours)

Week 1: Getting Started (Days 1-7)

8:00 AM: Break the fast with a nutrient-dense smoothie (spinach, kale, berries, Greek yogurt, chia seeds).

11:00 AM: Snack on a handful of almonds and an apple.

2:00 PM: Lunch with a quinoa salad (quinoa, cherry tomatoes, cucumber, avocado, baby spinach, olive oil, and lemon juice).

5:00 PM: Snack on baby carrots and hummus.

7:00 PM: Dinner with grilled chicken breast, quinoa, and steamed broccoli.

Week 2: Incorporating Variety (Days 8-14)

8:00 AM: Break the fast with avocado toast on whole grain bread, topped with a poached egg.

11:00 AM: Snack on Greek yogurt with a handful of berries.

2:00 PM: Lunch with a mixed greens salad (leafy greens, cherry tomatoes, cucumber, bell peppers, grilled chicken, olive oil, and balsamic vinegar).

5:00 PM: Snack on a small bowl of mixed nuts and an orange.

7:00 PM: Dinner with baked salmon, sweet potato, and sautéed spinach.

The 12:12 Kick-start 30-Day Plan

Week 3: Maintaining Momentum (Days 15-21)

8:00 AM: Break the fast with a smoothie bowl (blended berries, Greek yogurt, chia seeds, topped with granola and fresh fruit).

11:00 AM: Snack on a banana and a few slices of cheese.

2:00 PM: Lunch with a lentil and vegetable soup.

5:00 PM: Snack on an apple with a tablespoon of peanut butter.

7:00 PM: Dinner with beef stir-fry (grass-fed beef, bell peppers, broccoli, snap peas, and brown rice).

Week 4: Continuing Healthy Habits (Days 22-28)

8:00 AM: Break the fast with oatmeal topped with chia seeds, flaxseeds, and a handful of berries.

11:00 AM: Snack on cottage cheese with pineapple chunks.

2:00 PM: Lunch with a turkey and avocado wrap (whole grain tortilla, turkey slices, avocado, lettuce, tomato).

5:00 PM: Snack on sliced bell peppers with guacamole.

7:00 PM: Dinner with turkey meatballs, whole grain pasta, and marinara sauce.

The 12:12 Kick-start 30-Day Plan

Week 5: Final Week and Adjustments (Days 29-30)

8:00 AM: Break the fast with a nutrient-dense smoothie (spinach, kale, mango, Greek yogurt, chia seeds).

11:00 AM: Snack on a handful of walnuts and a pear.

2:00 PM: Lunch with a tofu and vegetable stir-fry.

5:00 PM: Snack on mixed berries and a small piece of dark chocolate.

7:00 PM: Dinner with stuffed bell peppers (bell peppers stuffed with ground turkey, brown rice, tomatoes, onions, and cheese).

_____

_____

_____

_____

Breaking the Fast: Tips and Adjustments

Regardless of whether you are doing 12:12 all the way to 16:8 then follows these general rules.

Start Gradually: Begin with small, nutrient-dense meals to avoid overwhelming your digestive system.

Hydrate: Drink water or herbal tea before breaking your fast to rehydrate.

Balanced Meals: Include proteins, healthy fats, and fiber in your meals to maintain energy levels and promote satiety.

Listen to Your Body: Adjust portion sizes and food choices based on how you feel. If you experience discomfort or digestive issues, consider lighter options like smoothies or soups.

Gradual Reintroduction: If taking a break from fasting after 30 days, gradually reintroduce a regular eating schedule to avoid shocking your system.

Finally, remember your nutrients.

Key Nutrients and Their Importance

Proteins: Essential for muscle repair and maintenance, helping preserve lean mass during fasting.

Carbohydrates: Focus on complex carbs like whole grains, fruits, and vegetables for sustained energy and digestive health.

Fats: Healthy fats from sources like avocados, nuts, and olive oil help with satiety, hormone production, and cellular health.

Vitamins and Minerals: Ensure intake of vitamins A, C, D, E, K, and B vitamins for immune function, skin health, and energy metabolism.

Fiber: Crucial for digestive health and managing blood sugar levels, found in whole grains, fruits, and vegetables.

By following this plan, you can support overall health, manage blood sugar levels, and maintain energy throughout your fasting and eating windows. Remember to listen to your body and adjust the plan as needed to ensure it meets your individual health goals and preferences.

Recipes

Here are seven recipes for the main meal in your intermittent fasting 12:12 diet plan:

Chapter 14

Moving up to 16:8 30 Day Plan

30-Day Meal Plan for a 16:8 Intermittent Fasting Diet

Like the 12:12 plan, and like the 13:11, 14:10, 15:9, the 16:8 30-day meal plan incorporates low and medium glycemic index (GI) foods, nutrient-dense ingredients, and vitamins and minerals

The main and only difference (to show you how easy it can be) is that the fasting window is smaller. In this example it is 8 hours. For other time-lengths where the fasting window is higher than 8 hours, simply adapt the meal and snack times.

Moving up to 16:8 30 Day Plan

Daily Structure

Fasting Window: 8:00 PM - 12:00 PM (16 hours)

Eating Window: 12:00 PM - 8:00 PM (8 hours)

Week 1: Getting Started (Days 1-7)

12:00 PM: Break the fast with a nutrient-dense smoothie (spinach, kale, berries, Greek yogurt, chia seeds).

3:00 PM: Snack on a handful of almonds and an apple.

6:00 PM: Dinner with grilled chicken breast, quinoa, and steamed broccoli.

7:30 PM: Snack on baby carrots and hummus.

Week 2: Incorporating Variety (Days 8-14)

12:00 PM: Break the fast with avocado toast on whole grain bread, topped with a poached egg.

3:00 PM: Snack on Greek yogurt with a handful of berries.

6:00 PM: Dinner with baked salmon, sweet potato, and sautéed spinach.

7:30 PM: Snack on a small bowl of mixed nuts and an orange.

Week 3: Maintaining Momentum (Days 15-21)

12:00 PM: Break the fast with a salad (leafy greens, cherry tomatoes, cucumber, bell peppers, grilled chicken, olive oil, and balsamic vinegar).

3:00 PM: Snack on a banana and a few slices of cheese.

6:00 PM: Dinner with beef stir-fry (grass-fed beef, bell peppers, broccoli, snap peas, and brown rice).

7:30 PM: Snack on an apple with a tablespoon of peanut butter.

Week 4: Continuing Healthy Habits (Days 22-28)

12:00 PM: Break the fast with oatmeal topped with chia seeds, flaxseeds, and a handful of berries.

3:00 PM: Snack on cottage cheese with pineapple chunks.

6:00 PM: Dinner with turkey meatballs, whole grain pasta, and marinara sauce.

7:30 PM: Snack on sliced bell peppers with guacamole.

Week 5: Final Week and Adjustments (Days 29-30)

12:00 PM: Break the fast with a nutrient-dense smoothie (spinach, kale, mango, Greek yogurt, chia seeds).

3:00 PM: Snack on a handful of walnuts and a pear.

6:00 PM: Dinner with baked tofu, quinoa, and roasted Brussels sprouts.

7:30 PM: Snack on mixed berries and a small piece of dark chocolate.

Chapter 15

Recipes

Recipes

Here are a weeks worth of recipes for the main meal in your intermittent fasting diet plan to get you started. These will work for any fasting window form 12 hours to 8 hours. Over the next week or two try to come up with your own using the nutrition and food information in chapters 5,6,7 and 8 (and make sure you are avoiding the 'bad' foods!).

1. Grilled Chicken Quinoa Bowl

Ingredients:

- 1 cup quinoa, rinsed
- 2 cups water or vegetable broth
- 2 chicken breasts, grilled and sliced
- 1 cup cherry tomatoes, halved
- 1 cucumber, diced
- 1 avocado, sliced
- 2 cups baby spinach
- 2 tbsp olive oil
- Juice of 1 lemon
- Salt and pepper to taste

Instructions:

In a medium pot, bring quinoa and water or broth to a boil. Reduce heat, cover, and simmer for 15 minutes, or until quinoa is cooked and water is absorbed. Fluff with a fork.

While quinoa is cooking, grill the chicken breasts until fully cooked, then slice them.

In a large bowl, combine cooked quinoa, cherry tomatoes, cucumber, avocado, and baby spinach.

Top with grilled chicken slices.

Drizzle with olive oil and lemon juice, and season with salt and pepper. Toss gently to combine and serve.

2. Baked Salmon with Sweet Potato and Asparagus

Ingredients:

- 2 salmon fillets
- 1 large sweet potato, peeled and cut into cubes
- 1 bunch asparagus, trimmed
- 2 tbsp olive oil
- 1 tsp garlic powder
- 1 tsp paprika
- Salt and pepper to taste
- Lemon wedges for serving

Instructions:

Preheat the oven to 400°F (200°C).

On a baking sheet, toss sweet potato cubes with 1 tbsp olive oil, garlic powder, paprika, salt, and pepper. Spread out in an even layer and bake for 15 minutes.

Remove the baking sheet from the oven and push the sweet potatoes to one side. Add the salmon fillets and asparagus to the baking sheet.

Drizzle the salmon and asparagus with the remaining olive oil and season with salt and pepper.

Return to the oven and bake for an additional 15-20 minutes, or until the salmon is cooked through and the sweet potatoes are tender.

Serve with lemon wedges.

3. Turkey Meatballs with Whole Grain Pasta

Ingredients:

- 1 lb ground turkey
- 1/4 cup breadcrumbs (whole grain if possible)
- 1/4 cup grated Parmesan cheese
- 1 egg
- 2 cloves garlic, minced
- 1 tsp dried oregano
- 1 tsp dried basil
- Salt and pepper to taste
- 1 tbsp olive oil
- 1 jar marinara sauce (low sugar)
- 8 oz whole grain pasta
- Fresh basil for garnish

Instructions:

In a large bowl, combine ground turkey, breadcrumbs, Parmesan cheese, egg, garlic, oregano, basil, salt, and pepper. Mix well and form into meatballs.

Heat olive oil in a large skillet over medium heat. Add the meatballs and cook until browned on all sides, about 8 minutes.

Add marinara sauce to the skillet, cover, and simmer for 15-20 minutes, or until meatballs are cooked through.

Meanwhile, cook the pasta according to package instructions. Drain and set aside.

Serve the meatballs and sauce over the pasta, garnished with fresh basil.

4. Beef Stir-Fry with Broccoli and Brown Rice

Ingredients:

- 1 lb beef sirloin, thinly sliced
- 1 tbsp soy sauce (low sodium)
- 1 tbsp oyster sauce
- 1 tbsp hoisin sauce
- 2 cloves garlic, minced
- 1 tbsp fresh ginger, minced
- 2 cups broccoli florets
- 1 red bell pepper, sliced
- 1 tbsp sesame oil
- 2 cups cooked brown rice
- Onions, sliced, for garnish
- Sesame seeds for garnish

Instructions:

In a bowl, mix soy sauce, oyster sauce, hoisin sauce, garlic, and ginger. Add the beef slices and marinate for at least 15 minutes.

Heat sesame oil in a large skillet or wok over medium-high heat. Add the marinated beef and stir-fry until browned, about 3-4 minutes.

Add broccoli and bell pepper to the skillet and stir-fry for another 5-7 minutes, until the vegetables are tender-crisp.

Serve the stir-fry over cooked brown rice, garnished with green onions and sesame seeds.

5. Lentil and Vegetable Curry

Ingredients:

- 1 cup red lentils, rinsed
- 1 onion, chopped
- 2 cloves garlic, minced
- 1 tbsp fresh ginger, minced
- 1 can coconut milk (13.5 oz)
- 1 can diced tomatoes (14.5 oz)
- 2 cups vegetable broth
- 1 tbsp curry powder
- 1 tsp turmeric
- 1 tsp cumin
- 1 tsp coriander
- 1 cup cauliflower florets
- 1 cup diced carrots
- 2 cups fresh spinach
- 2 tbsp olive oil
- Salt and pepper to taste
- Fresh cilantro for garnish

Instructions:

Heat olive oil in a large pot over medium heat. Add onion, garlic, and ginger and sauté until fragrant, about 5 minutes.

Add curry powder, turmeric, cumin, and coriander and cook for another 2 minutes.

Stir in lentils, coconut milk, diced tomatoes, and vegetable broth. Bring to a boil, then reduce heat and simmer for 15 minutes.

Add cauliflower and carrots, and simmer for another 10-15 minutes, or until vegetables and lentils are tender.

Recipes

Stir in spinach until wilted. Season with salt and pepper.

Serve with fresh cilantro on top.

6. Tofu and Vegetable Stir-Fry

Ingredients:

- 1 block firm tofu, drained and cubed
- 2 tbsp soy sauce (low sodium)
- 1 tbsp hoisin sauce
- 1 tbsp rice vinegar
- 1 tbsp sesame oil
- 2 cloves garlic, minced
- 1 tbsp fresh ginger, minced
- 1 red bell pepper, sliced
- 1 cup snap peas
- 1 cup broccoli florets
- 2 carrots, sliced
- 2 cups cooked quinoa
- Green onions, sliced, for garnish
- Sesame seeds for garnish

Instructions:

In a bowl, mix soy sauce, hoisin sauce, rice vinegar, garlic, and ginger. Add tofu cubes and marinate for at least 15 minutes.

Heat sesame oil in a large skillet or wok over medium-high heat. Add marinated tofu and stir-fry until browned, about 5-7 minutes. Remove tofu from skillet and set aside.

In the same skillet, add bell pepper, snap peas, broccoli, and carrots. Stir-fry for 5-7 minutes, or until vegetables are tender-crisp.

Return tofu to the skillet and toss to combine with vegetables.

Serve stir-fry over cooked quinoa, garnished with green onions and sesame seeds.

7. Stuffed Bell Peppers

Ingredients:

- 4 bell peppers, tops cut off and seeds removed
- 1 lb ground turkey or beef
- 1 cup cooked brown rice
- 1 can diced tomatoes (14.5 oz)
- 1 onion, chopped
- 2 cloves garlic, minced
- 1 tsp cumin
- 1 tsp paprika
- Salt and pepper to taste
- 1 cup shredded mozzarella or cheddar cheese
- 2 tbsp olive oil
- Fresh parsley for garnish

Instructions:

Preheat the oven to 375°F (190°C).
Heat olive oil in a large skillet over medium heat. Add onion and garlic and sauté until fragrant, about 5 minutes.
Add ground turkey or beef, cumin, paprika, salt, and pepper. Cook until meat is browned.
Stir in cooked brown rice and diced tomatoes. Simmer for 5 minutes.
Stuff the bell peppers with the meat and rice mixture. Place stuffed peppers in a baking dish.
Top each pepper with shredded cheese.
Cover with foil and bake for 30 minutes. Remove the foil and bake for an additional 10 minutes, or until the cheese is melted and bubbly.
Garnish with fresh parsley and serve

Date	Fasting Hours	Eating Window Start	Eating Window End	Foods consumed	Water Intake

Instructions:

- Document the start and end of your eating window each day.
- List all foods consumed during the eating window.
- Keep track of total water intake throughout the day.

Week ending date	Average Fasting Duration	Weight Change (if applicable)	Digestive Changes	Cognitive Changes	Emptional Changes	Skin Changes	Notes/ Reflections

Instructions:
- Note any reflections and/or summarize your observations and note any trends or significant changes.

Chapter 16

Your Fasting Lifestyle

Recommended Exercises

Engaging in regular physical activity is an essential component of a healthy lifestyle, particularly when combined with intermittent fasting. For individuals under 50, as well as men and women over 50, incorporating exercise can significantly enhance the benefits of fasting by improving overall health, boosting energy levels, and supporting metabolic function. Here are some recommended exercises that complement intermittent fasting and specifically address the needs of different age groups.

Under 50

Cardiovascular Exercises

Cardiovascular exercises, such as running, swimming, and cycling, are crucial for maintaining heart health and improving circulation. For those practicing intermittent fasting, engaging in moderate to high-intensity cardio can help enhance fat burning and improve insulin sensitivity. Running or jogging for 30-45 minutes a day can significantly boost cardiovascular health and stamina.

Strength Training

Strength training is vital for building and maintaining muscle mass, which supports metabolic health. Incorporating exercises like weightlifting, resistance band workouts, or bodyweight exercises (such as push-ups, squats, and lunges) can help build muscle and increase metabolic rate. For younger adults, integrating compound movements like deadlifts, bench presses, and pull-ups can maximize strength gains and muscle growth.

High-Intensity Interval Training (HIIT)

High-Intensity Interval Training (HIIT) involves short bursts of intense exercise followed by periods of rest or low-intensity exercise. HIIT can be an efficient way to boost metabolism and burn fat, even after the workout is completed. For those under 50, HIIT sessions can be particularly effective in enhancing fat loss and improving cardiovascular fitness. Exercises like sprinting, cycling, or bodyweight circuits (e.g., jumping jacks, burpees, and high knees) can be included in a HIIT routine. It is important to start slowly and gradually increase the intensity to avoid injury.

Women Over 50

Cardiovascular Exercises

Walking, swimming, and low-impact aerobics are excellent cardiovascular exercises for women over 50. These activities are gentle on the joints while effectively improving cardiovascular health. Engaging in these exercises for 30 minutes a day can enhance endurance and promote heart health.

Strength Training

Strength training becomes increasingly important as women age due to the natural decline in muscle mass and bone density. Incorporating light to moderate weightlifting, resistance band exercises, or bodyweight exercises (like modified push-ups, seated squats, and leg lifts) can help maintain muscle tone and support bone health. Weight-bearing exercises, in particular, are beneficial for preventing osteoporosis.

Flexibility and Balance Exercises

Yoga and tai chi are highly recommended for women over 50 to improve flexibility, balance, and reduce stress. These exercises enhance joint mobility and can help alleviate symptoms of menopause, such as mood swings and sleep disturbances. Gentle yoga poses and tai chi movements can be practiced daily to promote relaxation and overall well-being.

Men Over 50

Cardiovascular Exercises

For men over 50, incorporating cardiovascular exercises like brisk walking, swimming, or cycling can significantly improve heart health and stamina. These activities help reduce the risk of cardiovascular diseases and support weight management. Engaging in 30-45 minutes of cardio exercise most days of the week is beneficial.

Strength Training

Maintaining muscle mass is crucial for men over 50 to support metabolic health and overall strength. Incorporating moderate to heavy weightlifting with exercises like bench presses, rows, squats, and deadlifts can help preserve muscle mass and improve bone density. Strength training sessions should be performed two to three times a week, focusing on all major muscle groups.

Flexibility and Balance Exercises

Incorporating flexibility and balance exercises such as yoga or tai chi can enhance mobility and reduce the risk of falls. These exercises also help in managing stress and improving mental clarity. Simple stretches and balance exercises, like standing on one leg or practicing gentle yoga poses, can be done daily to improve flexibility and stability. It can be a great idea to do a yoga or tai chi routine with your partner.

Practical Implementation and Benefits

Combining different types of exercises ensures a well-rounded fitness routine that supports various aspects of health. Cardiovascular exercises improve heart health and endurance, strength training preserves muscle mass and boosts metabolism, and flexibility and balance exercises enhance mobility and reduce injury risk. For those practicing intermittent fasting, these exercises can significantly improve overall well-being and complement the metabolic benefits of fasting.

Engaging in regular physical activity while following an intermittent fasting regimen can lead to better health outcomes, increased energy levels, and enhanced physical and mental well-being. Whether you choose to walk, lift weights, practice yoga, the key is to find activities you enjoy and can sustain over the long term.

Other Lifestyle Practices

In addition to incorporating regular physical activity, there are several lifestyle practices that can significantly enhance the effects of intermittent fasting. These practices include stress reduction, adequate sleep, proper hydration, and mindful eating. Each of these components can play a role in maintaining overall health, particularly for individuals practicing intermittent fasting.

Stress Reduction

Stress reduction is essential for overall health and can significantly impact the effectiveness of intermittent fasting. Chronic stress can increase cortisol levels, which may lead to increased appetite and fat storage, particularly around the abdomen. Incorporating stress-reducing practices into your daily routine can help manage cortisol levels and improve overall health.

Meditation and Mindfulness: Practicing meditation and mindfulness can help calm the mind, reduce stress, and improve mental clarity. Spending even just 10-15 minutes a day in meditation can help lower cortisol levels and bring a sense of calm. Mindfulness practices, such as focusing on your breath or engaging in mindful eating, can also enhance your fasting experience.

Yoga and Tai Chi: Both yoga and tai chi are excellent for reducing stress and promoting relaxation. These practices combine gentle physical activity with deep breathing and meditative focus, which can help lower stress levels and improve overall well-being. Regular practice can enhance flexibility, balance, and mental clarity, making it easier to adhere to intermittent fasting routines.

Deep Breathing Exercises: Incorporating deep breathing exercises into your daily routine can help manage stress and improve respiratory function. Techniques such as diaphragmatic breathing or the 4-

7-8 breathing method can quickly reduce stress and promote relaxation. Practicing deep breathing for a few minutes each day can make a significant difference in your stress levels and overall health.

Adequate Sleep

Adequate sleep is crucial for overall health and well-being, and it significantly impacts the success of intermittent fasting. Poor sleep can disrupt hormonal balance, increase appetite, and reduce insulin sensitivity, making it harder to stick to a fasting schedule and achieve health goals.

Consistent Sleep Schedule: Establishing a regular sleep schedule by going to bed and waking up at the same time each day can improve sleep quality. Consistency helps regulate your body's internal clock, making it easier to fall asleep and wake up naturally.

Sleep Hygiene: Creating a restful sleep environment can enhance sleep quality. This includes keeping your bedroom cool, dark, and quiet, and avoiding screens (such as phones, computers, and TVs) at least an hour before bedtime. Engaging in a calming pre-sleep routine, such as reading a book or taking a warm bath, can also promote better sleep.

Limit Stimulants: Reducing the intake of stimulants such as caffeine and nicotine, especially in the hours leading up to bedtime, can improve sleep quality. Opting for caffeine-free herbal teas in the evening can be a soothing alternative.

Proper Hydration

Proper hydration is essential for overall health and supports the effectiveness of intermittent fasting. Dehydration can lead to fatigue, headaches, and decreased physical performance, making it harder to maintain fasting routines.

Signs of dehydration include dark urine, dry mouth, and dizziness. Keep a water bottle with you and set reminders to drink water if you find yourself not drinking enough to keep you properly hydrated.

Drink Plenty of Water: Aim to drink at least 8-10 glasses of water each day. Hydration helps flush out toxins, supports metabolic processes, and keeps your body functioning optimally. Starting your day with a glass of water and continuing to sip throughout the day can ensure you stay adequately hydrated.

Herbal Teas and Infusions: Herbal teas and infusions can be a great way to stay hydrated, especially during fasting periods. Teas such as chamomile, peppermint, and ginger can also help with things such as improved digestion and reduced inflammation.

Plain Black Coffee and Tea: Coffee and tea without any added sugar, milk, or cream is typically allowed. It can help with energy levels and may even enhance some of the benefits of fasting, such as fat burning and cognitive function.

Diluted Apple Cider Vinegar: Some people drink a small amount of apple cider vinegar diluted in water, as it may help with digestion and appetite control. Ensure it's well-diluted to avoid irritation.

Electrolyte Water: If you're engaging in prolonged fasting or exercising, an electrolyte drink without added sugars or calories can help maintain your electrolyte balance.

Bone Broth (longer fasts): For extended fasting periods (typically over 24 hours), some people drink bone broth to provide essential minerals and maintain electrolyte balance. Note that this is more applicable to longer fasts and may break a strict fast.

What to Avoid

Sugary Drinks: Any beverage with added sugars, including sodas, fruit juices, and sweetened teas or coffees, will break your fast.

Caloric Beverages: Drinks with calories, including milk, cream, and caloric sweeteners, should be avoided during the fasting window.

Alcohol: Alcoholic beverages should be avoided during fasting as they contain calories and can disrupt metabolic processes.

Mindful Eating

Mindful eating is a practice that involves paying full attention to the experience of eating and enjoying your food without distractions. This practice can improving digestion, promote better food choices, and helping you recognize hunger and fullness cues.

Eat Slowly: Taking your time to chew and savor each bite can improve digestion and help you feel more satisfied with your meals. This practice allows your body to properly signal when you are full, preventing overeating.

Focus on Nutrient-Dense Foods: During your eating windows, prioritize foods that are rich in nutrients. Incorporate a variety of fruits, vegetables, lean proteins, healthy fats, and whole grains into your meals. Nutrient-dense foods provide essential vitamins and minerals that support overall health and well-being.

Avoid Distractions: Eating without distractions, such as watching TV or using your phone, can help you fully enjoy your food and pay attention to your body's hunger and fullness signals. This can lead to more mindful eating habits and better portion control.

Goal Setting

Short-term: Start with intermittent fasting, identify personal health goals, and begin diversifying diet within a month.

What are the specific health benefits that you are seeking through fasting? Write your goals below.

Chapter Summary

Practical Diet Guide to Intermittent Fasting For Women Over 50

_____

_____

Long-term: Aim to establish a personalized and flexible fasting routine that matches your lifestyle and health goals over six months.

Begin thinking about this now and note any thoughts below.

Action Plan examples to support goals

Begin Intermittent Fasting: Start with a manageable fasting window, like 16:8, and gradually increase as comfortable.

Health Goal Identification: Write down specific health goals (weight loss, hormonal balance, etc.) and plan fasting types accordingly.

Dietary Diversification: Introduce new, healthy foods each week to support gut health and reduce cravings.

Building: Join or form a fasting support group for motivation and shared experiences.

Commitments: Schedule fasting times around personal and professional commitments for a balanced approach.

Lifestyle: Select 2 lifestyle approaches that you would like to explore with a view to adopting.

Hormonal Awareness: Track menstrual cycle (if applicable) and adapt fasting lengths to hormonal fluctuations.

Education and Self-Experimentation: Regularly read up on fasting and health topics, and experiment to find what works best.

Regular Review and Adjustment: Monthly check-ins to assess progress and make necessary adjustments to the fasting plan.

Embrace Setbacks as Learning Opportunities: Reflect on challenges faced and adapt strategies accordingly.

Sustain and Adapt: Continuously adapt the fasting routine to changing life circumstances and health needs.

Which of the above will you begin today? Pick 3 to get started.

Your Fasting Lifestyle

Chapter 17

Practical Tips and Tricks

Here are a few practical tips for enhancing the fasting experience including patience, practice, and learning.

But you will come across a few small hiccups along the way including how to manage hunger.

Understanding the underlying reasons for these strategies can help you make informed decisions and adapt fasting to your unique needs.

Managing Hunger During Fasting

Hunger and Boredom: One of the key challenges during fasting is distinguishing between true hunger and eating out of boredom. Emotional eating often stems from feelings of restlessness or boredom rather than any physical need. Try to find activities that occupy your mind and body, such as listening to music, reading or even dancing. Anything that can help you resist unnecessary cravings.

Electrolyte Balance: Electrolytes help maintain hydration and muscle function. During fasting, the body can lose essential minerals, which can lead to electrolyte imbalances. Using mineral supplements or electrolyte packets can help maintain your balance, which will also help to reduce hunger pangs, and prevent headaches or fatigue.

Beverage Choices While Fasting

Not all drinks are appropriate during fasting. Try to choose organic, herbal and pesticide-free coffee and tea which can prevent insulin resistance and support the fasting process.

Handling Detox Symptoms

Fasting can trigger detoxification, leading to symptoms such as the 'keto flu'. To manage these, vary your fasting routines and try methods like dry brushing or Epsom salt baths help with toxin elimination.

Dry brushing involves using a dry, stiff-bristled brush on the skin - typically done before bathing or showering, and performed on dry skin, not wet or damp. This technique has gained popularity for its potential health benefits, which include stimulating the lymphatic system, improving circulation, exfoliating the skin, and potentially reducing the appearance of cellulite.

Monitoring Blood Sugar and Ketones

Tracking Fasting: Monitoring your blood sugar and ketone levels can provide insights into the effectiveness of your fasting regimen. Tools like blood sugar and ketone meters offer instant readings, while Continuous Glucose Monitors (CGMs) provide detailed, real-time tracking of blood sugar levels. These tools help you understand how your body responds to fasting and make necessary adjustments.

Decreasing Blood Sugar

High blood sugar during fasting can slow or even stop progress. Again, mixing fasting routines, combined with a diet free of processed foods, can help insulin sensitivity and encourage ketosis. Make sure that your remember to monitor and make adjustments based on your body's responses - this is key to managing blood sugar levels effectively.

Fasting and Specific Conditions

Hair Loss During Fasting: One of the primary reasons for hair loss during fasting is a lack of essential nutrients. When fasting for extended periods, some people may not consume enough vitamins and minerals required for healthy hair growth leading to nutritional deficiencies which can affect the hair growth cycle, leading to hair thinning and loss. A doubly whammy because menopause can also impact hair loss,

You can help this by shortening your fasting window or considering some of these vitamins and supplements.

1. Zinc: Zinc is vital for hair tissue growth and repair. It helps keep the oil glands around the hair follicles working properly. A deficiency in zinc can lead to hair loss and a dry, flaky scalp.

Sources: Meat, shellfish, legumes, seeds, nuts, dairy, eggs, and whole grains.

2. Iron: Iron deficiency is a common cause of hair loss, particularly in women. Iron is essential for red blood cells to transport oxygen to cells, including hair follicles.

Sources: Red meat, poultry, fish, lentils, spinach, and fortified cereals.

3. Magnesium: Magnesium plays a role in various biochemical reactions in the body, including those involved in hair growth. It helps in protein synthesis and the formation of strong hair strands.

Sources: Nuts, seeds, whole grains, leafy green vegetables, and fish.

4. Selenium: Selenium is important for the proper functioning of the thyroid gland, which regulates metabolism and affects hair growth. It also has antioxidant properties that protect hair follicles from damage.

Sources: Brazil nuts, seafood, eggs, and sunflower seeds.

5. Biotin (Vitamin B7): Biotin is crucial for hair health, as it supports the production of keratin, a protein that makes up hair, skin, and nails. A deficiency in biotin can lead to hair thinning and loss.

Sources: Eggs, nuts, seeds, sweet potatoes, and spinach.

6. Vitamin D: Vitamin D plays a role in creating new hair follicles and is important for hair growth. Low levels of vitamin D have been linked to alopecia, a condition that causes hair thinning and loss.

Sources: Fatty fish, fortified foods, beef liver, cheese, and egg yolks. Sun exposure also helps the body produce vitamin D.

Fatigue and Sleep

Fatigue is another common issue during fasting while sleep quality can be affected too - which doesn't help fatigue! Supplements such as magnesium or CBD can help you sleep better or you can try red light therapy to boost energy levels.

Overcoming Challenges in Fasting

Taking breaks from fasting is natural, but resuming can sometimes be challenging. Adopting a non-judgmental attitude and easing back into fasting gradually can help you regain momentum without stress.

Key Takeaways

The fasting journey is a personal and evolving process that can require patience and persistence.

Understanding that healing and results take time, especially for chronic conditions, is crucial.

Approach fasting as a skill that improves with practice, and don't be discouraged by setbacks.

Continuously educating yourself about fasting and varying your fasting routines can prevent adaptation and stalling progress.

Employing detoxification techniques and handling special conditions with care can enhance the benefits of fasting.

A mindful approach, being aware of your body's signals

Avoid fasting during sensitive periods like pregnancy and nursing.

By managing hunger, choosing suitable beverages, handling detox symptoms, and monitoring key health indicators, you can optimize the benefits of fasting.

Practical Diet Guide to Intermittent Fasting For Women Over 50

Reflective Questions:

How can you differentiate between true hunger and boredom during your fast?

What strategies can you use to gradually increase your fasting duration?

How can you incorporate fasting into your routine while addressing specific health conditions you have?

In what ways can you educate yourself more about the benefits and processes of fasting?

How can you ensure that your fasting practice is helping, not harming, your overall health and well-being?

Goal Setting

Short-Term Goal: Start with intermittent fasting, aiming for a 13-hour fast, and gradually increase the duration over the next month.

Long-Term Goal: Develop a personalized fasting routine that fits your health needs and lifestyle, aiming for consistent practice over six months.

Action Plans

Begin Intermittent Fasting: Start with a manageable fasting period and slowly extend it, paying attention to your body's response.

Monitor Health Metrics: Regularly check blood sugar and ketone levels to assess the effectiveness of your fasting.

Incorporate Detox Methods: Include practices like dry brushing and adequate hydration to support detoxification.

Educate Yourself: Watch informational videos and join online communities to deepen your understanding of fasting.

Consult Health Professionals: Discuss your fasting plans with a healthcare provider, especially if you have specific health conditions.

Getting Started

The following pages provide a place to begin. First, set you goals and action plan then use the example logs and planners to get you started in developing your own unique fasting plan.

Chapter 18

5 Key Goals

5 Short Term Goals

----

5 Long-term Goals

_____

_____

_____

_____

_____

Chapter 19

Action Plans

Use this section to review the action plans that you have thought about over the course of this workbook.

Write the action plans that meet your long and short term goals.

Action plan to reach your short term goals

Action Plans

Select 5 of the most important actions for your short-term goals

_____

_____

_____

_____

_____

Action plan to reach your long-term goals

Action Plans

Select 5 of the most important actions for your long-term goals

---

Chapter 20

Beginner Fasting Logs

In the next pages there are two ways and sets of tables to keep track of your fasting and how you feel. Try them out and decide on the best type of tracker for you.

The first set are split into Fasting and Nutrition, Physical and Emotional Wellbeing, and Health Metrics and Obervations.

Use these tables as a guide for logging your fasting. Each page has 7 days. If you are doing a 30 day fast then use the same format for 30 days.

Here are the primary aspects to monitor:

Fasting Duration: Record the start and end times of each fasting period. This will help you maintain consistency and observe patterns over time. For intermittent fasting like 16:8, note the time window you are eating and the time you are fasting.

Dietary Intake During Eating Windows: Log what you eat during non-fasting periods, focusing on the quality and quantity of food. This is crucial to ensure that you're getting the necessary nutrients and not overeating after a fast.

Physical Responses: Keep track of any physical changes or symptoms you experience, such as energy levels, sleep quality, digestive changes, and any signs of discomfort or unusual bodily responses.

Emotional and Mental Well-being: Fasting can impact your mood and mental state. Record any significant changes in your emotional well-being, mental clarity, or stress levels.

Weight and Body Measurements (if applicable): If weight management is a goal, regularly track your weight and possibly other body measurements like waist circumference.

Hydration Levels: Ensure you're drinking enough water and staying hydrated, especially during fasting periods. Tracking your water intake can be helpful.

Menstrual Cycle (for women): Women should pay special attention to their menstrual cycle, noting any changes in cycle regularity, duration, or symptoms, as fasting can affect hormonal balance.

Sleep Patterns: Monitor your sleep quality and duration, as fasting can sometimes influence sleep.

Physical Activity Levels: Record your exercise routines as they may need to be adjusted according to your fasting schedule

Blood Glucose and Ketone Levels (if applicable): For those following a ketogenic approach or managing conditions like diabetes.

Subjective Well-being: Keep a journal or notes on how you feel overall while fasting. This can include levels of hunger, energy, focus, and general well-being.

Medical Check-ups and Lab Tests (if necessary): If you have pre-existing health conditions or if you're undertaking long-term fasting, regular medical check-ups and lab tests (like lipid profiles, liver function tests, etc.) can be important to ensure that the fasting regime is not adversely affecting your health.

By tracking these elements, you can gain a better understanding of how fasting affects your body and mind, make necessary adjustments, and ensure a safe and effective fasting experience. Remember, individual responses to fasting can vary significantly, so what works for one person may not work for another. It's always advisable to consult with a healthcare provider before starting any new diet, especially if you have pre-existing health conditions.

Select 5 of the most important parts of you daily routine that are foundational to begin change and add the time at which they take place

----

Begin by creating your daily plan for the next 7 days. You can download a 30 day plan here or simply copy the headings onto a blank journal.

Fasting and Nutrition

Date	Fasting Start Time	Fasting Duration	Food Consumed (During Eating Window)	Water Intake

Physical and Emotional Wellbing

Date	Physical Symptonms (Energy, Digestion etc)	Emotional Mental State	Sleep Quality	Exercise Activity

Health Metrics & Observations

Date	Weight/ Body Measure-ments	Mentrual Cycle Notes (if applicable)	Blood Glucose, Ketone Levels (if applicatbe)	General Wellbing Notes

Weekly beginner logs

The second set of log tables for fasting cover a week at a time. There are 3 tables which make up your week and four sets of these logs.

You can mix and match both types of tables to find the one that works best for you and that meets your needs.

Date	Fasting Hours	Eating Window Start	Eating Window End	Foods consumed	Water Intake

Instructions:

- Document the start and end of your eating window each day.
- List all foods consumed during the eating window.
- Keep track of total water intake throughout the day.

Date	Energy Level (1-10)	Mental Clarity (1-10)	Digestive Health (1-10)	Digestive Health (1-10)	Mood (1-10)	Physical Acitivty (1-10)	Sleep Quality incl Hrs (1-10)	Unusual Symptoms	Overall Well-being (1-10)

Instructions:
- Rate your energy levels, mental clarity, digestive health, mood, and overall well-being on a scale of 1 to 10.
- Note the type and duration of physical activity.
- Record sleep duration and quality, along with any unusual symptoms you might experience.

Week ending date	Average Fasting Duration	Weight Change (if applicable)	Digestive Changes	Cognitive Changes	Emptional Changes	Skin Changes	Notes/ Reflections

Instructions:
- Note any reflections and/or summarize your observations and note any trends or significant changes.

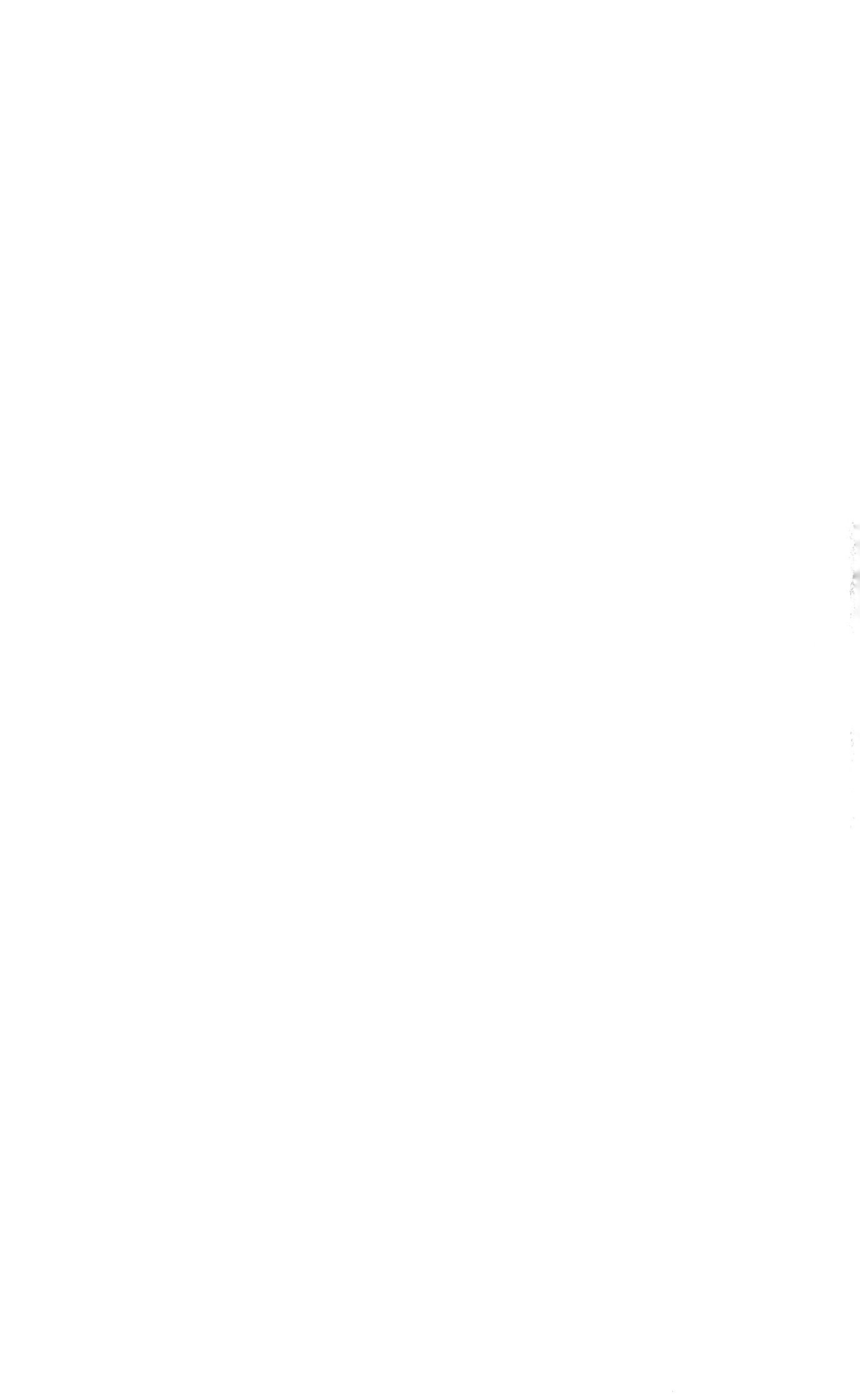

Date	Fasting Hours	Eating Window Start	Eating Window End	Foods consumed	Water Intake

Instructions:
- Document the start and end of your eating window each day.
- List all foods consumed during the eating window.
- Keep track of total water intake throughout the day.

Date	Energy Level (1-10)	Mental Clarity (1-10)	Digestive Health (1-10)	Digestive Health (1-10)	Mood (1-10)	Physical Acitivty (1-10)	Sleep Quality incl Hrs (1-10)	Unusual Symptoms	Overall Well-being (1-10)

Instructions:
- Rate your energy levels, mental clarity, digestive health, mood, and overall well-being on a scale of 1 to 10.
- Note the type and duration of physical activity.
- Record sleep duration and quality, along with any unusual symptoms you might experience.

Week ending date	Average Fasting Duration	Weight Change (if applicable)	Digestive Changes	Cognitive Changes	Emptional Changes	Skin Changes	Notes/ Reflections

Instructions:
- Note any reflections and/or summarize your observations and note any trends or significant changes.

Date	Fasting Hours	Eating Window Start	Eating Window End	Foods consumed	Water Intake

Instructions:
- Document the start and end of your eating window each day.
- List all foods consumed during the eating window.
- Keep track of total water intake throughout the day.

Date	Energy Level (1-10)	Mental Clarity (1-10)	Digestive Health (1-10)	Digestive Health (1-10)	Mood (1-10)	Physical Acitivty (1-10)	Sleep Quality incl Hrs (1-10)	Unusual Symptoms	Overall Well-being (1-10)

Instructions:

- Rate your energy levels, mental clarity, digestive health, mood, and overall well-being on a scale of 1 to 10.
- Note the type and duration of physical activity.
- Record sleep duration and quality, along with any unusual symptoms you might experience.

Week ending date	Average Fasting Duration	Weight Change (if applicable)	Digestive Changes	Cognitive Changes	Emptional Changes	Skin Changes	Notes/ Reflections

Instructions:
- Note any reflections and/or summarize your observations and note any trends or significant changes.

Date	Fasting Hours	Eating Window Start	Eating Window End	Foods consumed	Water Intake

Instructions:
- Document the start and end of your eating window each day.
- List all foods consumed during the eating window.
- Keep track of total water intake throughout the day.

Date	Energy Level (1-10)	Mental Clarity (1-10)	Digestive Health (1-10)	Digestive Health (1-10)	Mood (1-10)	Physical Acitivty (1-10)	Sleep Quality incl Hrs (1-10)	Unusual Symptoms	Overall Well-being (1-10)

Instructions:
- Rate your energy levels, mental clarity, digestive health, mood, and overall well-being on a scale of 1 to 10.
- Note the type and duration of physical activity.
- Record sleep duration and quality, along with any unusual symptoms you might experience.

Week ending date	Average Fasting Duration	Weight Change (if applicable)	Digestive Changes	Cognitive Changes	Emptional Changes	Skin Changes	Notes/ Reflections

Instructions:
- Note any reflections and/or summarize your observations and note any trends or significant changes.

Chapter 21

Conclusion

It's clear that intermittent fasting offers a multitude of benefits for individuals over 50, and indeed for people of all ages and it's more than diet; it's a sustainable lifestyle change that can lead to improved health, greater vitality, and enhanced longevity.

Intermittent fasting can help regulate blood sugar levels, improve insulin sensitivity, and reduce the risk of type 2 diabetes. By incorporating fasting into your routine, you can better manage your metabolic health and maintain a healthy weight. By reducing your eating window, you naturally consume fewer calories, which can aid in weight loss and prevent weight gain. The flexibility of intermittent fasting allows you to choose a schedule that fits your lifestyle, making it easier to stick with in the long term.

Chronic inflammation is a common issue that can lead to various health problems. Intermittent fasting helps reduce inflammation, promoting better overall health and reducing the risk of chronic diseases. Many people report increased energy levels and mental clarity as a result of intermittent fasting. This is due to more stable blood sugar levels and improved metabolic function.

Conclusion

Fasting triggers autophagy, a natural process that cleans out damaged cells and promotes the regeneration of healthy cells. This cellular rejuvenation can slow down the aging process and improve overall health. Intermittent fasting is flexible and can be adapted to fit your personal needs and lifestyle. Whether you start with a 12:12 plan and progress to a 16:8 schedule, or find another pattern that works for you, the key is consistency and listening to your body.

Intermittent fasting is a powerful tool that can help you achieve better health, more energy, and a greater sense of well-being. By embracing this lifestyle, you are taking a proactive step towards improving your quality of life. Remember that the journey to health is personal and unique to each individual. Be patient with yourself, stay informed, and enjoy the process of discovering what works best for you.

As you move forward, use the knowledge and strategies you've gained from this book to create a fasting plan that fits seamlessly into your life. Whether you continue with a 12:12 schedule, progress to a 16:8 plan, or find another pattern that suits you, the important thing is that you are making choices that support your health and longevity.

Here's to a healthier, happier, and more vibrant life!

Chapter 22

References

SM Muscat, RM Barrientos - Experimental gerontology, 2020 - Elsevier. Lifestyle modifications with anti-neuroinflammatory benefits in the aging population. nih.gov

M Pereira, J Liang, J Edwards-Hicks, AM Meadows... - Cell reports, 2024 - cell.com. Arachidonic acid inhibition of the NLRP3 inflammasome is a mechanism to explain the anti-inflammatory effects of fasting. cell.com

G Kenđel Jovanović, I Mrakovcic-Sutic, S Pavičić Žeželj... - Nutrients, 2020 - mdpi.com. The efficacy of an energy-restricted anti-inflammatory diet for the management of obesity in younger adults. mdpi.com

Madeo, F., & Kroemer, G. (2020). "Fasting and caloric restriction in cancer prevention and treatment." Nature Reviews Cancer, 20(2), 74-75.

Ristow, M., & Schmeisser, S. (2014). "Mitohormesis: Promoting health and lifespan by increased levels of reactive oxygen species (ROS)." Dose-Response, 12(2), 288-341. Link

References

Sun, N., Youle, R. J., & Finkel, T. (2016). "The Mitochondrial Basis of Aging." Molecular Cell, 61(5), 654-666. Link

Mrazek, A. A., & Talley, N. J. (2017). "Fasting and Gut Microbiota: Effects on Gastrointestinal Health." Gastroenterology Clinics of North America, 46(1), 69-83. Link

Longo, V. D., & Panda, S. (2016). "Fasting, circadian rhythms, and time-restricted feeding in healthy lifespan." Cell Metabolism, 23(6), 1048-1059. Link

Mattson, M. P., & Arumugam, T. V. (2018). "Hallmarks of brain aging: Adaptive and pathological modification by metabolic states." Cell Metabolism, 27(6), 1176-1199. Link

Rothman, S. M., & Mattson, M. P. (2013). "Activity-dependent, stress-responsive BDNF signaling and the quest for optimal brain health and resilience throughout the lifespan." Physiology & Behavior, 122, 20-29.

Cryan, J. F., & Kaupmann, K. (2005). "GABAB receptors: A new focus in antidepressant drug discovery." Current Drug Targets-CNS & Neurological Disorders, 4(5), 579-592.

Voisin, S., Eynon, N., Yan, X., & Bishop, D. J. (2015). "Exercise training and DNA methylation in humans." Acta Physiologica, 213(1), 39-59.

Angelopoulos, T. J., Foulis, S. A., & Metzler, J. N. (2018). The impact of intermittent fasting on health and disease. *Journal of the Academy of Nutrition and Dietetics*, 118(4), 747-753. https://doi.org/10.1016/j.jand.2017.10.024

Hunt, N. D., Hyun, D. H., Allard, J. S., Minor, R. K., Mattson, M. P., Ingram, D. K., & de Cabo, R. (2006). Bioenergetics of aging and calorie restriction. *Ageing Research Reviews*, 5(2), 125-143. https://doi.org/10.1016/j.arr.2006.02.005

Knüsel, M., Mohajeri, M. H., & Niggli, U. A. (2015). Effect of selenium and zinc supplementation on hair growth in healthy individuals with low hair density. *Journal of Trace Elements in Medicine and Biology*, 29, 253-257. https://doi.org/10.1016/j.jtemb.2014.07.013

Lichtenstein, A. H., Appel, L. J., Brands, M., Carnethon, M., Daniels, S., Franch, H. A., ... & Van Horn, L. (2006). Diet and lifestyle recommendations revision 2006: a scientific statement from the American Heart Association Nutrition Committee. *Circulation*, 114(1), 82-96. https://doi.org/10.1161/CIRCULATIONAHA.106.176158

Mason, J. B. (2011). Vitamins, trace minerals, and other micronutrients. In M. H. Manson (Ed.), *Textbook of Clinical Nutrition and Functional Medicine* (Vol. 2, pp. 173-189). Manson Publishing.

Pilkington, K., Kirkwood, G., Rampes, H., Richardson, J., & Charandabi, S. (2005). Yoga for depression: the research evidence. *Journal of Affective Disorders*, 89(1-3), 13-24. https://doi.org/10.1016/j.jad.2005.08.013

Song, Y., & Manson, J. E. (2008). Magnesium intake and bone mineral density in women. *Journal of the American College of Nutrition*, 27(2), 245-252. https://doi.org/10.1080/07315724.2008.10719697

Zempleni, J., & Mock, D. M. (1999). Biotin biochemistry and human requirements. *Journal of Nutrition*, 129(2), 485-487. https://doi.org/10.1093/jn/129.2.485S

Pilkington, K., Kirkwood, G., Rampes, H., Richardson, J., & Charandabi, S. (2005). Yoga for depression: the research evidence. *Journal of Affective Disorders*, 89(1-3), 13-24. https://doi.org/10.1016/j.jad.2005.08.013

American Dietetic Association. (2009). Position of the American Dietetic Association: Nutrition and lifestyle for a healthy pregnancy outcome. *Journal of the American Dietetic Association*, 109(5), 918-927. https://doi.org/10.1016/j.jada.2009.03.008

References

Mattson, M. P., Moehl, K., Ghena, N., Schmaedick, M., & Cheng, A. (2018). Intermittent metabolic switching, neuroplasticity and brain health. *Nature Reviews Neuroscience*, 19(2), 63-80. https://doi.org/10.1038/nrn.2017.156

National Institutes of Health. (2019). Zinc: Fact Sheet for Health Professionals. https://ods.od.nih.gov/factsheets/Zinc-HealthProfessional/

Rautiainen, S., Manson, J. E., Lichtenstein, A. H., & Sesso, H. D. (2016). Dietary supplements and disease prevention – A global overview. *Nature Reviews Endocrinology*, 12(8), 407-420. https://doi.org/10.1038/nrendo.2016.54

Schwalfenberg, G. K. (2011). A review of the critical role of vitamin D in the functioning of the immune system and the clinical implications of vitamin D deficiency. *Molecular Nutrition & Food Research*, 55(1), 96-108. https://doi.org/10.1002/mnfr.201000174

Harvard T.H. Chan School of Public Health - The Nutrition

National Institutes of Health (NIH) - Cellular Health

National Institute of Diabetes and Digestive and Kidney Diseases (NIDDK) - Understanding Metabolism

American Diabetes Association - Insulin Resistance

World Health Organization (WHO) - Obesity and Food Quality

Environmental Working Group (EWG) - Obesogens

Mayo Clinic - Stress Management

Office on Women's Health (OWH) - Hormonal Health

Frontiers in Oncology, 2023

https://my.clevelandclinic.org/health/diseases/22206-insulin-resistance

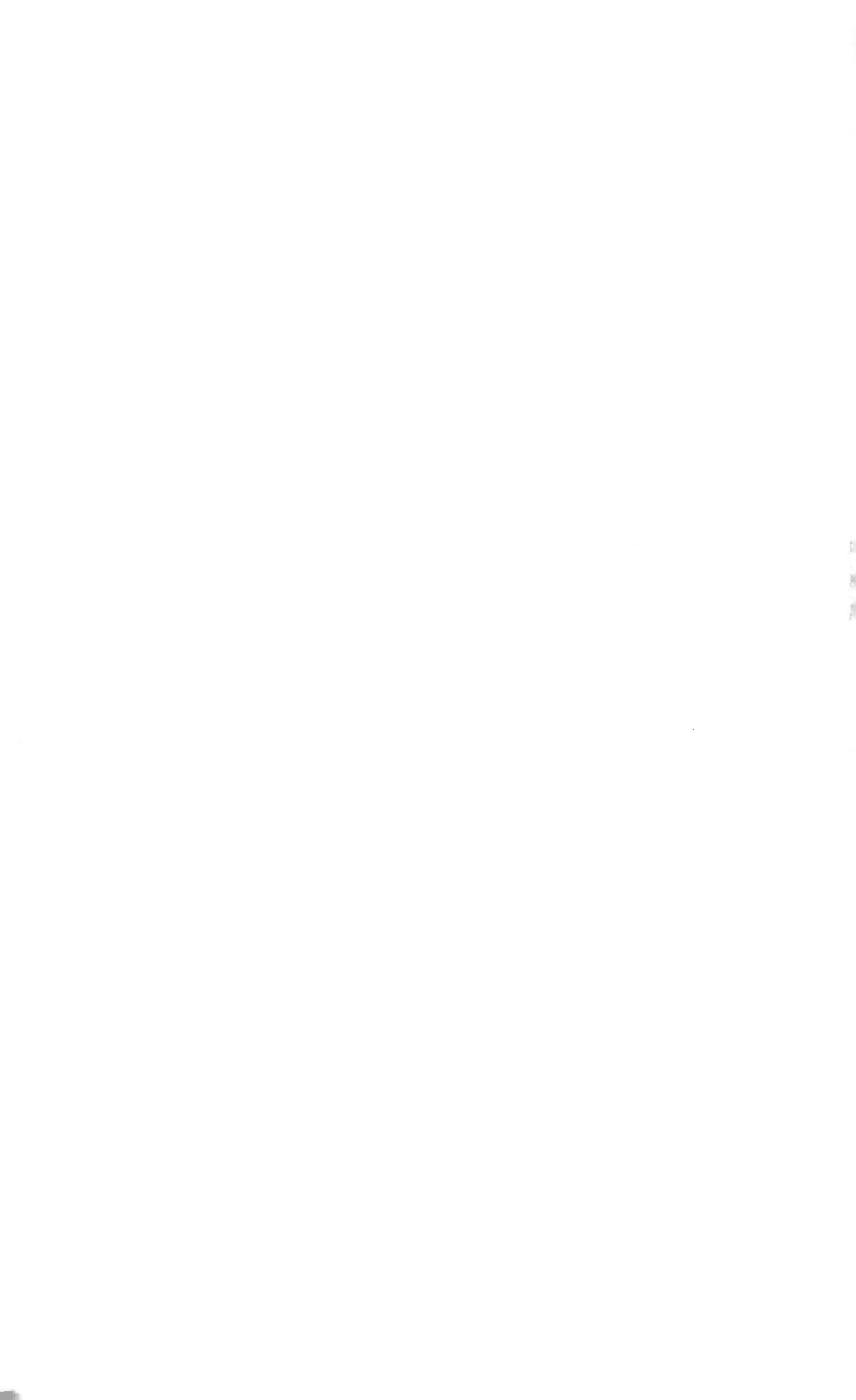

Printed in Great Britain
by Amazon

52092118R00137